Health, Illness, and Disability in Later Life

SAGE SOURCEBOOKS FOR
THE HUMAN SERVICES SERIES

Series Editors: ARMAND LAUFFER and CHARLES GARVIN

Recent Volumes in this Series

Rosalie F. Young
Elizabeth A. Olson
editors

Health, Illness, and Disability in Later Life

Practice Issues and Interventions

SAGE SOURCEBOOKS FOR THE HUMAN SERVICES SERIES 17

SAGE PUBLICATIONS
The International Professional Publishers
Newbury Park   London   New Delhi

For information address:

SAGE Publications, Inc.
2455 Teller Road
Newbury Park, California 91320

SAGE Publications Ltd.
6 Bonhill Street
London EC2A 4PU
United Kingdom

SAGE Publications India Pvt. Ltd.
M-32 Market
Greater Kailash I
New Delhi 110 048 India

Printed in the United States of America

Library of Congress Cataloging-in-Publication Data

Health, illness, and disability in later life : practice issues and
   interventions / edited by Rosalie F. Young and Elizabeth A. Olson.
       p. cm. — (Sage sourcebooks for the human services series ;
  v. 17)
   Includes bibliographical references.
   Includes index.
   ISBN 0-8039-3965-5 — ISBN 0-8039-3966-3 (pbk.)
   1. Aged—Health and hygiene.   I. Series.
   [DNLM: 1. Aging. 2. Chronic Disease—in old age. 3. Family.
  4. Health Services for the Aged. 5. Mental Health—in old age. WT
  100 H4334]
  RA564.8.H426   1991
  613'.0438—dc20
  DNLM/DLC
  for Library of Congress   90-9222
                                               CIP

FIRST PRINTING, 1991

Sage Production Editor: Judith L. Hunter

CONTENTS

Part I

HEALTH, ILLNESS, AND DISABILITY IN LATER LIFE: CONCERNS FOR PRACTITIONERS

INTRODUCTION

ROSALIE F. YOUNG
ELIZABETH A. OLSON

OVERVIEW OF HEALTH AND DISEASE
IN LATER LIFE

Today, a typical 65-year-old individual can expect to survive 17 more years and live an active life in the community until well into his or her seventies. If this person is a woman, she can expect to live, on the average, to be 84 years old. Although a 65-year-old man is likely to survive only 15 more years, he still will live beyond the "three score and ten" indicator of longevity. Indeed, when we examine death figures in the late 1980s we see that a rectangular survival pattern is increasingly common. Rather than a steadily increasing death rate from childhood on with a downward sloping line (the common pattern for the 1840s), Fries and Crapo (1985) have shown that a large portion of the population lives to be almost 80. After that time death rates increase significantly, resulting in a rectangularization of the mortality pattern. Thus, by eliminating many causes of preventative death, there is almost a right angle of mortality.

Table A

Rates Per 1,000 Persons Age 65 and Older for Selected Chronic Conditions, 1984

Arthritis	490
Hypertension	406
Heart	320
Diabetes	103
Bronchitis	63
Ulcer	33

SOURCE: National Center for Health Statistics, 1985.

As we consider these formidable trends toward longer life, it is essential to couple this knowledge with realization of the fact that many of our steadily increasing population of 30 million older persons have important health needs. Close to 90% of older persons have chronic conditions, many of which are quite serious. To illustrate, there are 11 million hypertensives, more than 4 million heart patients, and 3 million diabetics who are age 65 or older. We also find that ulcers and respiratory problems afflict significant numbers of older people. In 1984, rates for major chronic conditions were quite high among the elderly (See Table A). Furthermore, there is a tendency for many older persons to have multiple chronicities, meaning that they are afflicted with two or more chronic conditions simultaneously.

As serious as these trends may be (for example, approximately one half of older persons have arthritis and half are hypertensive), they mask the significant increase in chronic-disease death and disability that occurs with each additional decade of life after age 65. For example, we find that persons aged 85 and older died of coronary heart disease at the rate of 7,000 per 100,000 in 1984, a figure seven times greater than that of persons 65-74 (National Center for Health Statistics, 1985). When we couple these facts with the startling population increase projected for the age 85 and over cohort (they presently number more than two million and will show a sevenfold increase by 2050), it is increasingly clear that illness and disability at later life will increase.

We should keep in mind that most of the aged are living in their communities. At any given point in time, only 5% reside in nursing homes. However, the nursing home population is expected to triple to 4.5 million in 2040. Perhaps of greater salience is the fact that the lifetime risk of nursing home placement is over 40% (Liu, Manton, & Liu, 1985) and, while many of the elderly will spend only a short time in nursing homes, for women over the age of 85 the likelihood of nursing home placement is extremely high. This group is not only very likely to be physically frail, but mental health and cognitive functioning problems also are common. Furthermore, even among older women with few physical limitations, the lack of a spouse, small size of social networks, and low income level combine to make them a great risk for nursing home placement. They may not be seriously impaired or unable to care for themselves, but because they cannot attend to home management needs or are unable to shop or do their laundry, they may ultimately need nursing home care.

There are many misconceptions about the mental status of older persons. Most community-living elderly have satisfactory to excellent levels of cognitive functioning. Only 9% of persons over the age of 65 are seriously impaired with regard to thinking and remembering. Most elders in this category suffer from Alzheimer's disease or serious physical diseases that reduce oxygen flow to the brain. Foremost among these are strokes or congestive heart failure. The mental status decline of many physically ill elders exemplifies that aging and disease are distinct bodily processes. Whereas aging predisposes the body to disease states (for example, the aging musculoskeletal system causes bone to be more brittle and fractures more common), old does not necessarily mean ill, any more than ill means old. With regard to thinking, learning, and remembering, older people with certain types of physical health problems are much more likely to be cognitively impaired than their healthy counterparts.

These trends and figures are quite important for persons serving the elderly in a variety of health and human service fields. Few practitioners can afford to ignore problems that are raised by the prevalence of illness and disability in later life. This is particularly the case when we consider chronic disease among older persons.

Chronic conditions, such as those listed in Table A, exact tolls in several areas. Certainly they affect adversely the health and functioning of the stricken individual. There are effects well beyond those that apply only to older patients, however. As this volume will show in later chapters, lingering and/or serious health problems place major burdens on the ailing individual, his or her family and community, and the health care services of that community. With regard to the older patient, he or she often is adversely affected in areas that extend considerably beyond basic health and functioning. There are consequences for the older person's psychological, social, and economic functioning. The patient's family and significant others also are affected by illness situations, particularly serious chronic conditions such as heart attack or those that cause a high degree of functional impairment such as arthritis. The family has a major role to play in illness, and the family-illness intermesh in later life is complex. Communities and society also are affected and the impact can be quite negative. There is a significant drain upon medical and economic resources related to providing health care for ailing aged. Furthermore, social and human service agencies often must intervene to assist the chronically ill or frail aged in a variety of ways. Three areas need to be addressed. First, that the health problems of the older segment of our society will continue to grow in number and scope. Second, that there will be need for a major increase in hospital and long-term care facilities and additional numbers and types of health providers to treat these problems. Third, communities will need to address the services that can best benefit the ailing elderly and their families who often are faced with informal caregiving activities.

IMPLICATIONS OF LATE-LIFE HEALTH PROBLEMS FOR PRACTITIONERS

Whatever our field of practice, the prevalence of health problems—especially those pertaining to chronic disease of the aged—requires our utmost attention. We need to consider the facts themselves and also the necessity for professional intervention. The facts are described briefly above; intervention is the focus of this volume. There are certain broad needs and effects that have an impact on both facts and intervention. Briefly discussed below, these needs are to consider the impact of late-life illness on the patient or client; to consider familial and societal effects of late-life illness; to develop multidisciplinary approaches to intervention; and to improve skills and knowledge for professional intervention with the elderly.

Considering the Impact on Patient and Client

Later life illness has many aftereffects. The physical reserve of the elderly is much less than that of their younger counterparts and recuperation is slower. There is much greater likelihood of medical complications of health problems and greater risk of secondary involvement. Mental health issues can arise.

Those who work with the elderly recognize the important interface between physical and mental health at later life. Disease states reduce physical capacity and increase the need for assistance. Dependency states may result. These situations are very distressing to the elderly. Thus it is not uncommon to note that morale and general life satisfaction lessen among physically ailing elders. Illness also taxes the coping responses of the aged and often generates anxiety, depression, and emotional strain. There are many mental health effects that have little direct relationship to the health problem but are secondary effects of the patient's interpretation of his or her disability.

Social functioning also is affected in adverse ways. Clearly, lingering chronic conditions affect activity levels and social participation. Physically demanding activities often must be eliminated and general social participation may decline. Basic interaction with family and friends is changed and may be significantly reduced. The chronically ill older person may become increasingly socially isolated. Obviously, this affects his or her general morale. Hence, we often see spiraling aftereffects of a major enduring health problem.

Considering Familial and Societal Effects

The family-illness intermesh is particularly apparent in later life. There are mutual effects of illness upon the family system. Similarly, the family system can have significant impact upon the health status of the patient.

With regard to the former, health problems place care provision and psychological burdens upon those who are closely involved with the ailing person. Reassuring or comforting the older patient also become tasks of family and friendship networks. Caregiving is a major family function and most elderly and their children alike expect to experience this situation. As chapters in this book will show, neither is happy with the situation, but both adjust as best they can.

The family also can exert considerable influence upon the illness itself. An activist family may cooperate with physicians and insure compliance with recommendations, organize caregiving among many individuals, access formal support systems, communicate effectively and often with medical personnel, and engage in many activities that facilitate recovery or aid recuperation. Families also can act in ways that impede recovery or exacerbate the health problem. Nevertheless, few elders experience illness without involving their family and kinship networks in the process.

Health problems of the aged impinge upon a community's medical, financial, institutional, and human resources. For example, heart disease accounts for more usage of health care services than any other condition of the elderly; 20% of the hospital stays of persons over age 65 are due to heart conditions. The cost of treatment for heart disease alone is expected to increase almost 50% in the next 25 years, according to recent estimates of the National Center for Health Services Research and Health Care Technology Assessment.

Health problems of the elderly presently require health and human service provision at many levels of expertise. A variety of services and institutions presently are serving the ailing aged. In the future, however, society may find that the health needs of the elderly exceed resources. Few communities will be able to ignore such needs, and society will be pressed for ways to provide personnel and facilities to serve the ailing aged in effective and economical ways. Rather than continuing with our present system of care, which is costly and still unable to deliver the necessary services to the ailing aged, communities may incorporate the principles of a "continuum of care." A range or continuum of in-home, congregate living, and facility-centered services will need to be available to deal with the health-generated needs of the aged.

Multidisciplinary Approaches to Intervention

Health and aging are closely interrelated. As discussed earlier, chronic illnesses affect many aspects of the lives of older individuals in addition to health status, such as psychological, social, and economic functioning. The goal of most interventions is to assist the older person to "age in place," that is, to maintain the individual in his or her own home as long as possible and to avoid institutionalization.

Achievement of this goal requires intervention that recognizes the impact of chronic illness on the older patient's or client's everyday life and that represents a variety of disciplines. Professionals need to give attention to the whole of the older person's life and to all the factors that complete its context (including the social, psychological, and economic) as well as to the presenting symptoms.

The primary objective of this book is to examine intervention approaches from a variety of disciplines. The book is divided into several parts, each exploring different aspects of illness, disability, and health in later life and describing intervention strategies aimed at assisting older adults to maintain independence as long as possible.

Improving Skills and Knowledge for Professional Intervention

There is a continuing and growing need for current, research-based, and policy-informed information for health and human service providers assisting older adults. In order to provide the best assistance and to help as many older adults as possible, service providers—both health professionals and social services professionals—need to have a basic understanding of the issues and concerns of the elderly and of new and improved methods of assistance.

As the population rapidly grows older, the knowledge base concerning aging also is growing at a quick pace. Research on all aspects of aging and the characteristics of the aged is being conducted, with important and practice-relevant findings being reported daily. Because the study of the processes of aging is multidisciplinary in perspective, new information is being developed in many different fields concurrently. Improved diagnostic and care-provision techniques are being developed constantly. Public policies affecting the elderly and their families are being modified continually and new policies and programs initiated. With information regarding aging growing so rapidly, service providers need to keep abreast of subject matter related to services they provide, such as new resources that may benefit the older adults they serve. This volume offers practical suggestions for implementing both current intervention approaches and professional development programs.

PRIORITY AREAS FOR INTERVENTION

As the contributors to this volume show, there are several areas of intervention that can help to ameliorate the problems discussed above. Some require very focused, intense interventions. Others can be helped with more general strategies. Still others require the involvement of persons with many types of expertise and will not be possible without a multidisciplinary approach.

The authors contributing to this volume have addressed the areas of the biological aspects of aging, health and medical concerns, mental health issues, problems of alcohol abuse, violence against the elderly, and family implications of illness. The issues addressed are directly approached by the authors. The chapters represent a combination of clinical skills and practical advice. Each author has bridged the gap of research and application with concrete suggestions.

REFERENCES

Fries, J. F., & Crapo, L. M. (1985). The elimination of premature disease. In K. Dychtwald (Ed.), *Wellness and health promotion*. Denver, CO: Aspen.

Liu, K., Manton, K. G., & Liu, B. (1985). Home care for the disabled elderly. *Health Care Financing Review, 2*, 51-58.

National Center for Health Statistics. (1985). *Health, U.S.* (DHHS Publications No. PHS 86-1232). Washington, DC: Government Printing Office.

Part II

HEALTH OF THE ELDERLY: STATUS, BEHAVIORS, AND RISKS

Chapter 1

MODIFYING THE AGING PROCESS

ROBERT ARKING

Why would we want to modify the aging process? The question almost seems to answer itself. Most of us, probably even all of us, would prefer to live as long as we can, provided that our lives are more than just some minimal physical existence supported by tubes and hospital heroics. As the saying goes, there should be some life in our years. But few would object if the years were more instead of less. Obviously, the wish for a "magic potion" or a fountain of youth did not die with Ponce de Leon but persists among us even in this transmuted form. Perhaps each of us would like to live longer, or at least age slower, than most of our fellow travelers. How can we do that? Is it even possible? What is the stuff that dreams are made of and where do we get some of it for ourselves?

A decade or two ago, there would have been no good answer to this fundamental biological question. Today, however, we are in a position to amalgamate recent advances made in the basic biology of aging—data obtained from both animal and human studies—which when taken together present a very plausible and maybe even a probable answer to these not so frivolous questions. Actually the question we posed to ourselves above has two parts: (a) Can we slow down the rate of aging and, if so, what does this

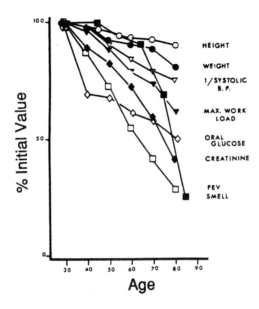

Figure 1.1. The Changes in Various Physical Functions and Attributes with Age

NOTE: The mean values for 30 year olds are taken as 100% and subsequent scores are normalized to this value. The decrements shown are schematic linear projections that emphasize the overall trend while omitting the variability. The height, weight, and creatinine clearance are taken from longitudinal studies.

SOURCE: R. Arking (1990).

mean to each of us; and (b) Is there an inherent limit to the human life span and, if so, what does this mean to each of us? Let us deal with each of these questions separately.

SLOWING THE RATE OF AGING

We can measure the rate of aging by determining the change in various physiological functions with age. A compilation of such measurements drawn from a variety of studies is shown in Figure 1.1.

These data show that both anatomical measurement and physiological functions decrease with age. Clearly, these functional decreases underlie the aging process and provide the intimate physical failings with which each of us are only too familiar. Of course, there exists a great deal of variance between individuals that is not shown in these data, but this does not obscure or alter the overall trend. Given this situation, we would want to pursue those biological strategies that either would (a) arrest the decline in function or (b) at least slow down the rate of decline. The idea here of course is that both the quantity and quality of our years is related to our physiological states. If we can age successfully, then we can remain healthy for a long time and enjoy the benefit of our years. The challenge facing us is that we would like to be able to functionally measure the aging process and selectively intervene in such a way so as to retard the loss of physiological function—to deliberately make ourselves age more slowly. Clearly, we can absorb substantial decrements in our various physiological functions without adversely affecting our ability to function under normal circumstances. What is affected, however, is our reserve capacity. We become more and more susceptible to dying from a stress that would hardly have bothered us when we were younger.

THE LIMITS TO LIFE

The second question had to do with whether or not there is an inherent and rigid limit to the human life span. If there is, then that would set fixed constraints on the limits of whatever interventions we might devise. If the human life span is somewhat plastic, however, then our interventions might be more successful than we might even dare dream. The place to look for the answer is in the human survival data covering this century, the time span during which we have seen very large and meaningful increases in the life span (see Figure 1.2).

We can see that there have been large increases (approximately 41%) in the mean life span between 1900 and 1980, coupled with relatively small increases (approximately 8%) in the maximum life span during this same time period. The increases in the mean life expectancy have been largely brought about by dramatic decreases in the incidence of premature or nonsenescent deaths among the young and, more recently, among the middle aged (Myers & Manton, 1984). The changes in the maximum life span, however, are well within the accepted maximum value of 120 years for the human species. Thus it is quite possible that the increase in these maximum ages is more apparent than real; they might simply be statistical quirks. If so, then perhaps there are real limits to the life span.

Do such limits exist? Perhaps Woody Allen said it for all of us: "Some people want to achieve immortality through their works or their descendants. I prefer to achieve immortality by not dying." Well, is his wish even theoretically possible? There are science fiction writers who think so, but what of reality? Is this a future option? Probably not. The nearest you and I can come to measuring immortality is to measure the life span of some

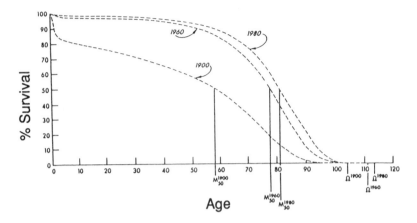

Figure 1.2. Mortality Survival Curves for U.S. Females in 1900, 1960, and 1980
NOTE: The M50 line marks the median age at death, and the M100 symbol marks the maximum age at death, for each of these three populations. The 1900-1960 interval was marked by rapid declines in infant and child mortality, while the 1960-1980 interval is characterized by declines in (primarily cardiovascular) mortality at later ages. The significant gains in life expectancy, obtained by overcoming the causes of premature death, do not appear to inhibit the progression toward increased survival, even today.
SOURCE: G. C. Myers & K. G. Manton (1984). Reprinted by permission.

inanimate object that does not have to put up with the insults and injuries of living. Brown and Flood (1947) measured the life span of glass tumblers used in a cafeteria and guess what happened: even inanimate objects cannot live forever simply because accidents happen. No matter how long you live, you will eventually die, if only from an accident. Nothing is forever.

FUTURE OPTIONS

We only have three possible future options. One option is that the future shall resemble the past, that the aging process is immutable, and there is nothing we can do to alter our fates. I do not believe that the actual data supports this pessimistic point of view. The choice between the next two options rests on whether or not the human life span has a fixed limit of about 120 years as implied by the maximum life span data of Figure 1.2. If it does, then the best we can hope for is to drastically slow down the rate of aging so that we all stay healthy throughout 98% of our life and then, at the very end, die quickly and easily of some system failure. In effect, we will have discovered how to take the senescent diseases that now afflict our last 15 or 20 years and compress them into the last year or so of our life. This is popularly known as "rectangularizing the curve" (Fries & Crapo, 1981). The data of Figure 1.2 offer no support for the existence of this process (Myers & Manton, 1984). The third option is based on the assumption that the human life span does not have a rigidly fixed limit. If this assumption can be verified by hard data, then our third option suggests that we might be able to significantly increase both mean and maximum life spans without, however, abolishing senescent diseases. In effect, we will have discovered how to extend our middle adult years without significantly affecting the course of our eventual senescence. Let us examine the data regarding both of these questions.

Measuring Aging: The Use of Biomarkers

How do we know if we have modified the aging process? You might say that if someone lives to be 150 or so then it is reasonable to conclude that they did something right. Well, yes, that might provide good tales for reporters and tourists, but it just won't do for serious biogerontology work. First, such an approach has severe conceptual faults, not the least of which is the fact that it depends entirely upon retrospective evidence. Second, such descriptive and anecdotal evidence can be very misleading. Much was printed in the popular press a few decades ago about superlong-lived people leading a primitive life-style in the Caucasus or in the Andes, living until the age of 165 years or so. Unfortunately, research has shown that these tales are just that and their anecdotal claims of having significantly extended the maximum human life span have no basis in fact (Leaf, 1985; Medvedev, 1986). Finally, this and other such incidents has made us realize that chronology may not be the best way to measure aging. We have all known or heard about pairs of individuals, both of whom are about the same chronological age but are of vastly different functional ages. It is not the number of their years that distinguishes them but rather the level of their performance. If we want to measure the changes in our physiology with aging so that we can determine whether or not some intervention has successfully modified the aging process, then what we need is some functional marker.

A biological marker of aging, or biomarker for short, has been defined as an important biological or behavioral function that is altered with aging; that is not susceptible to major influences by environmental factors, and that may serve to measure the rate of physiological aging. One can assay age according to three somewhat different standards (Walford, 1986). First would be those biomarkers that defined one's functional or intrinsic age at the time of testing. Examples of these would include vital capacity, maximal oxygen capacity, kidney function, visual accommodation, and the like. Next are those

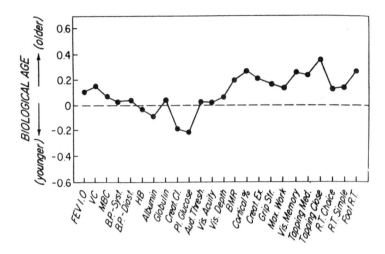

Figure 1.3. Biological Age Profile of a Single Individual Based on the Indicated Biomarkers.

NOTE: The dotted line represents the mean score for this person's age group for each of the indicated biomarkers. This profile demonstrates that an individual may be biologically older on some parameters than others, and that a normal individual may deviate quite strikingly from the mean.

SOURCE: G. A. Berkan & A. H. Norris (1980). Reprinted by permission.

biomarkers that can be used to predict one's remaining life expectancy, barring accidents. Examples of these would include immune-function tests, systolic blood pressure, reaction time, and hand grip strength. Finally, there exists a class of biomarkers which, although rather susceptible to environmental influence (such as diet and exercise), are still valuable in highlighting a susceptibility to a particular disease, possibly because of an accelerated aging of one particular organ system. Examples of this last class would include blood cholesterol levels and the LDL/HDL ratios, glucose-tolerance, and so forth. It should be noted that there do exist certain cogent objections to any extensive theoretical reliance on these biomarkers, particularly since our current knowledge of the aging process is still fragmentary and it is difficult to decipher the causal or correlative relationship of any given biomarker to the basic aging processes involved (Costa & McCrae, 1985).

The concept of biomarkers and their usefulness has been demonstrated in studies such as the Baltimore Longitudinal Study on Aging (Shock et al., 1984). Figure 1.3 presents the results of some 24 different physiological functions as measured in one individual from the BLSA study. These data illustrate the mosaic nature of aging and show that the individual's chronological age alone is a very poor predictor of his or her organ-specific

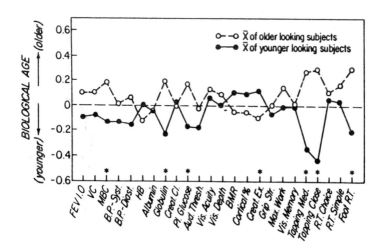

Figure 1.4. Biological Age Profile of Two Populations Based on Their Subjectively Estimated Age.

NOTE: The open circles represent the mean biological age scores of individuals in the subpopulation that appeared most "old for their age" (top 15% of distribution). The solid circles represent the mean biological age scores of individuals in the subpopulation that appeared most "young for their age" (bottom 15% of population). The asterisks indicate parameters for which the difference between the two groups was statistically significant.

SOURCE: G. A. Borkan & A. H. Norris (1980). Reprinted by permission.

functional age. Individuals participating in the BLSA were divided subjectively by the physicians into two discrete populations; those who looked older than their ages and those who looked younger than their ages. When their summed biomarker scores were compared, it was found that the older looking individuals tended to have older biomarker scores (Figure 1.4). When a similar procedure was done with BLSA participants, only this time comparing the most recent scores of the living and the dead BLSA subjects, the biomarker scores diverged in the expected direction. All this suggests (but does not prove) that biomarkers are probably measuring some functionally important aspects of the aging processes and that the choice of the right biomarkers might provide us with a quantitative measure of functional aging.

What does all this mean in terms of our initial questions? The Duke Longitudinal Study (Palmore, 1981) measured the effects of a series of physical and socioeconomic factors on the longevity of its subjects. The study examined the effects of a number of social, economic, cultural, behavioral, and physiological factors on the longevity of its participants. The researchers concluded that, statistically, the health of the individual was the most important predictor. It logically follows that our biomarker profile of our health is perhaps the most important (but not the only) factor controlling our own personal aging rate. Thus it might prove possible to use them as objective, physiologically valid, organ-specific, nonchronological markers of aging.

Intervening in Aging

Now that we can begin to see just how we can functionally measure the aging process, what can we do to modify the aging process? It turns out that substantial progress has been made in answering this question and that there is room for guarded optimism. There are but two proven methods of modifying aging and longevity. These are (a) genetic manipulation and (b) nutritional interventions.

Genetic Manipulations

Genealogical studies have been done on humans, thanks to our propensity for detailed record keeping, and they all agree with the interpretation that our heredity plays a major role in determining, and is a good predictor of, our life span. Experimental genetic studies have all, for obvious reasons, been done on animals (most particularly the mouse), on common bread mold, and on insects such as the fruit fly and the uncommon nematode (something like a very small "worm"). Scientists study such diverse and odd species for a variety of reasons, not the least of which is the particular suitability of that particular animal for that particular question. Are the differences between the different species important? Of course they are, but they are probably less important than we might think. As we shall see, genetically based extensions of life span have been reported in fungi, flies, worms, and mice. These different species might well accomplish this alteration by different mechanisms. The real import of these findings is that they make it very clear that our own maximum life span is not irreversibly encoded along our DNA but can be experimentally manipulated and extended. Let us quickly review some of these pertinent results.

In the nematode, genetic mutants have been sought and found that exhibit significant extensions of the life span, ranging up to a 70% increase in both the mean and the maximum values (Johnson, 1987).

In the common bread mold, *Neurospora,* it has proven possible to use artificial selection to increase the mean and maximum life span by 300% or to decrease them by 50% (Munkres & Furtek, 1984).

In the fruit fly, *Drosophila,* we have been able to bring about a 50% increase in the mean and maximum life span by means of artificial selection

(Arking, 1987), while Grigliatti (1987) has isolated a mutation that accelerates the normal aging process and thereby reduces the life span values.

In the common house mouse, there exist many inbred strains, almost all of which have been bred for characteristics other than aging and longevity. Nonetheless, a comparison of their life span data indicates that their hereditary differences cause them to have widely different longevities (Goodrich, 1975). The longer-lived strains have a 20% increase in their mean life span over the comparable values for the ordinary strains, while the shorter-lived strains show a 60% decrease in their mean life span over the ordinary values. The short-lived strains do not age faster but they do seem to be very susceptible to certain degenerative diseases and die prematurely. They might be viewed as being comparable to short-lived human families with histories of early onset heart disease. It is possible that the long-lived strains may age more slowly than average, as shown by their biomarker data and by the absence of any specific pathologies assigned as a cause of death.

These experimental data clearly show that there probably is not a rigidly fixed limit to these species' specific maximum life spans. In at least these four diverse species, genetic manipulation appears to have reconstructed the bodily physiology so as to slow down the rate of aging and greatly increase the mean and maximum life span. It is likely that the genetic processes involved act so as to delay the onset of certain key physiological events and thereby slow down the rate of aging. There probably is some sort of eventual intrinsic limit to life span but the data suggest that limit has not yet been reached in at least these species. We know or suspect three more things about this genetic effect. First, it is likely that the genes in at least two of these species may be affecting the antioxidant enzymes, such as superoxide dismutase or catalase, which protect us from the harmful effects of oxygen. Second, there are a surprisingly small number of genes involved in the regulation of longevity, ranging from one in the worm to perhaps six or so chromosomal regions/genes in the mouse and the fly (Gelman, Watson, Bronson, & Yunis, 1988; Johnson, 1987). Third, all of the human and animal data support the view that longevity is a genetically determined, environmentally modulated process that is best measured by the passage of particular physiological events.

Nutritional Interventions

There is, however, one major problem with such data. It is all very well to manipulate the genomes of experimental animals; it is quite another thing to do that with humans. Much more practical would be the development of some kind of nongenetic intervention that would be reasonable for individual

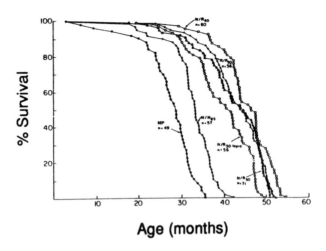

Figure 1.5. Survival Curves of Mice Fed Various Diets

NOTE: Each symbol represents an individual mouse. Note the large changes in both the mean and maximum life-span values. Diet groups are as follows: NP—standard lab chow fed *ad libitum*; N/N85—mice fed *ad libitum* with a purified diet after weaning at about 50 kcal. per week; N/R 50 lopro—as before but with dietary protein content decreasing with age; N/R 40--mice fed a restricted diet after weaning at about 40 kcal. per week; R/R40—mice fed a restricted diet both before and after weaning at about 40 kcal. per week.

SOURCE: R. Weindruch, R. L. Walford, S. Fligiel, & D. Guthrie (1986). Reprinted by permission.

people to use or not, as they choose. Does such a choice even exist? Yes, it does, and it is called nutritional intervention.

This does not refer to the normal sorts of urging we hear from our physicians and our nagging relatives to slim down, not eat junk food, lose weight, or look better. It is related to the ordinary sorts of dieting but is distinctly different, for the goal is not weight loss as a result of temporary dieting per se but rather a *permanent* caloric restriction.

This line of investigation began more than a half century ago when Clive McKay and associates (1935) studied the effects of food deprivation in rats. He observed that food restriction beginning at weaning resulted in extraordinarily long-lived rats. The diet was so strict that the animals effectively stopped growing unless their caloric intake was increased. Furthermore, this dietary regime also gave rise to some pretty stupid rats as well as to some nonproducing rats as a result of protein deprivation. The intervention obviously was not suitable for use in people. The basic findings were confirmed over the years but remained only as a laboratory curiosity. Starting about a decade or so ago, it was reinvestigated, using different types of dietary regimes. The data in Figure 1.5 (Weindruch, Walford, Fligiel, & Guthrie,

1986) illustrate that when the mice's postweaning diet is adjusted so that there is no deficiency in any of the essential nutrients but only a permanent deficiency in their caloric intake, major increases in the mean and the maximum life spans are observed.

A diet in which the caloric intake is reduced to about 60% of the control value yields about a 30% increase in the mean and maximum life spans. A more stringent diet in which the caloric intake is reduced to about 47% of the control value yields about a 35% increase in the mean and maximum life span values. Of course, if one compares the restricted animals to the ad libitum fed (NP) group, then the increase in life span approaches 50%. It should not escape our attention that the effect of dietary manipulation on the life span parameters is comparable to those achieved by the genetic manipulations. Furthermore, caloric restriction is effective in mice even when started in mid-adult life (Weindruch & Walford, 1982). In such situations, the increase in life span is reduced proportionately to the time when the caloric restriction was started.

Just what is it that caloric restriction is doing and how does it relate to what we know about the biology of the aging process? The first thing to realize is that it is not determined by how fat an individual is. When genetically obese mice are put onto a caloric restriction regime, they also live an extraordinarily long time though their bodily fat content still remains two to four times higher than the normal values (Harrison, Arder, & Astle, 1984). They are still fat, but they live as long as do the normal diet-restricted animals. Other studies have shown that it is not due to animals eating an excess of protein, or fat, or carbohydrates, or any other single component of the diet, nor is it due to the elimination of some toxic component from the diet (Masoro, 1988). It seems simply to be due to a reduction of the total amount of food eaten—a reduction in the total amount of calories taken in. A close inspection of Figure 1.5 will bear this out. No formal diet restriction experiments have been conducted on humans, for obvious reasons. Yet the absence of such data cannot be construed as evidence in favor of a rigidly fixed human life span, especially since the informal human data that is available is consistent with the conclusions drawn from animal studies. Current thinking, based on much data that will not be examined here (but see Everitt, 1982; Finch, 1987; or Richardson et al., 1985, for review and references) suggests that caloric restriction affects gene activity via its effects on the neuroendocrine system and eventually on hormone-dependent gene action in a variety of other tissues. Another equally plausible suggestion is that the caloric restriction results in the decreased production of harmful by-products of metabolism, by-products that are thought to damage the cell and possibly underlie the physiological decrements characteristic of aging (Weindruch et al, 1986).

The animal studies unequivocally tell us two things: (a) genetic manipulation can bring about a slower rate of aging and an increased longevity, and (b) caloric restriction can bring about a slower rate of aging and an increased longevity. They also suggest that we might want to rethink just what constitutes optimal nutrition for humans.

Practical Applications of Theoretical Knowledge

No one wants to have his or her genes tampered with, even if we knew what to do, which we do not, so this option does not even exist for us at the present time. Our only remaining option, if we wish to modify our rate of aging, is to practice permanent caloric restriction. This raises a problem of implementation. People in our society have great difficulty in eating less and losing weight even when their reasons for doing so are quite pressing and pertinent to their everyday needs and wishes. This task is so difficult that many of us spend good money and precious time to join diet and health groups or to buy the newest diet book. It is probably unrealistic to expect many of our neighbors and friends (much less ourselves) to suddenly change their ways and uncharacteristically elect to initiate and follow the stringent diet regimes dictated by the animal studies. Nobody wants to be on a perpetual diet. So what is an ordinary person with ordinary frailties to do?

Roy Walford has developed the High-Low diet program as a partial answer to this problem. The name derives putting together a diet that is high in nutritional value and low in caloric content. His program consists of much more than just a diet, for it involves monitoring your own biomarkers while losing weight very gradually over a five-year period. It is fully described in his book (Walford, 1986), which should be read for a more detailed discussion of the program. It should be noted that you might profit from monitoring your own biomarkers even if you do not go on the diet. It has been pointed out that there exists a positive relationship between one's health and one's sense of control, and that this relationship is mediated through known physiological mechanisms (Rodin, 1986). Following this program, even in part, may give one a psychological boost and have a health-enhancing effect over and above the purely physiological aspects examined in the animal studies.

This idea of a permanent caloric restriction is not a fad type of idea. Caloric restriction is an idea that was discovered in the lab 50 years ago and has been tested through a variety of stringent experiments. It is now recognized as the only effective method of manipulating the aging rate in mammals. The current interest in this intervention manifests itself in various ways, all of which suggests that this intervention is now being examined for its practical utility. The process is currently being prepared to be moved out of the laboratory and into the world.

SUMMARY

In conclusion, this rapid survey of recent advances in the biology of aging shows that aging is a genetically determined, environmentally modulated process that is best measured by the passage of particular physiological events rather than by the passage of time. In the laboratory, it has proved possible to genetically manipulate various experimental species so as to significantly extend both the mean and the maximum life spans. This agrees with human studies showing that our heredity plays a major role in determining our longevity. Various environmental interventions have been examined in the laboratory, of which the most strikingly successful is that of caloric restriction. Monitoring our caloric intake, along with monitoring our biomarkers, allows individuals to exert some significant control over their own aging process.

REFERENCES

Arking, R. (1987). Successful selection for increased longevity in Drosophila: Analysis of the survival data and presentation of a hypothesis on the genetic regulation of longevity. *Experimental Gerontology, 22,* 199-220.

Arking, R. (1990). *Biology of the aging: Observations and principles.* Englewood Cliffs, NJ: Prentice-Hall.

Borkan, G. A., & Norris, A. H. (1980). Assessment of biological age using a profile of physical parameters. *Journal of Gerontology, 35,* 177-184.

Brown, G. W., & Flood, M. M. (1947). Tumbler mortality. *Journal of the American Statistical Association, 42,* 562.

Costa, P. T., Jr., & McCrae, R. R. (1985). Concepts of functional or biological age: A critical view. In R. Andres, E. L. Bierman, & W. R. Hazzard (Eds.), *Principles of geriatric medicine.* New York: McGraw-Hill.

Everitt, A. V. (1982). Nutrition and the hypothalamic-pituitary influence on aging. In G. B. Moment (Ed.), *Nutritional approaches to aging research.* Boca Raton, Florida: CRC Press.

Finch, C. E. (1987). Neural and endocrine determinants of senescence: Investigation of causality and reversibility by laboratory and clinical interventions. In H. R. Warner, R. N. Butler, R. L. Sprott, & E. L. Schneider (Eds.), *Modern biological theories of aging* (Vol. 31). New York: Raven.

Fries, J. M., & Crapo, L. M. (1981). *Vitality and aging: Implications of the rectangular curve.* San Francisco: Freeman.

Gelman, R., Watson, A., Bronson, R., & Yunis, E. (1988). Murine chromosomal regions correlated with longevity. *Genetics, 118,* 693-704.

Goodrich, C. L. (1975). Life span and inheritance of longevity of inbred mice. *Journal of Gerontology, 30,* 257-263.

Grigliatti, T. A. (1987). Programmed cell death and aging in Drosophila melanogaster. In A. D. Woodhead & K. H. Thompson (Eds.), *Evolution of longevity in animals: A comparative approach.* New York: Plenum.

Harrison, D. E., Arder, J. R., & Astle, C. M. (1984). Effects of food restriction in aging: Separation of food intake and adiposity. *Proceedings of the National Academy of Sciences, 81,* 1835-1838.

Johnson, T. E. (1987). Aging can be genetically dissected into component processes using long-lived lines of Caenorhabditis elegans. *Proceedings of the National Academy of Sciences, 84,* 3777-3781.

Leaf, A. (1985). Long-lived populations (extreme old age). In R. Andres, E. L. Bierman, & W. R. Hazzard (Eds.), *Principles of geriatric medicine.* New York: McGraw-Hill.

Masoro, E. J. (1988). Food restriction in rodents: An evaluation of its role in the study of aging. *Journal of Gerontology: Biological Science, 43,* B59-B64.

McKay, C. M., Crowell, M. F., & Maynard, L. A. (1935). The effect of retarded growth upon the length of the life span and upon ultimate body size. *The Journal of Nutrition, 10,* 63-79.

Medvedev, Z. A. (1986). Age structure of Soviet population in the Caucasus: Facts and myths. In A. H. Bittles & K. J. Collins (Eds.), *The biology of human aging.* Cambridge: Cambridge University Press.

Munkres, K. D., & Furtek, C. A. (1984). Selection of conidial longevity mutants of Neurospora crassa. *Mechanisms of Aging and Development, 25,* 47-62.

Myers, G. C., & Manton, K. G. (1984). Compression of mortality: Myth or reality. *The Gerontologist, 24,* 346-353.

Palmore, E. (1981). *Social patterns in normal aging: Findings from the Duke longitudinal study.* Durham, NC: Duke University Press.

Richardson, A., Rutherford, M. S., Birchenall-Sparks, M. C., Roberts, M. S., Wu, W. T., & Cheung, H. T. (1985). Levels of specific messenger RNA species as a function of age. In R. S. Sohal, L. S. Birnbaum, & R. G. Cutler (Eds.), *Molecular biology of aging: Gene stability and gene expression* (Vol. 29). New York: Raven.

Rodin, J. (1986). Aging and health: Effects of the sense of control. *Science, 233,* 1271-1276.

Shock, N. W. (1972). Energy metabolism, caloric intake and physical activity of the aging. In L. A. Carlson (Ed.), *Nutrition in old age: X Symposium Swedish Nutrition Foundation.* Uppsala, Sweden: Almqvist & Wiksell.

Shock, N. W., Greulich, R. C., Costa, R. T., Jr., Andres, R., Lakatta, E. G., Arenberg, D., & Tobin, J. D. (1984). *Normal human aging: The Baltimore longitudinal study of aging* (NIH Publication No. 84-2450). Washington, DC: Government Printing Office.

Walford, R. (1986). *The 120 year diet: How to double your vital years.* New York: Pocket Books.

Weindruch, R., & Walford, R. (1982). Dietary restriction in mice beginning at 1 year of age: Effect on life span and spontaneous cancer incidence. *Science, 215,* 1415-1418.

Weindruch, R., Walford, R. L., Fligiel, S., & Guthrie, D. (1986). The retardation of aging in mice by dietary restriction: Longevity, cancer, immunity and lifetime energy intake. *The Journal of Nutrition, 116,* 641-654.

Chapter 2

HEALTH PROMOTION AND RISK REDUCTION FOR LATER LIFE

JOSEPH W. HESS

The notion that it is worthwhile and potentially cost-effective to attempt to reduce the risk of disease and disability in older adults is of relatively recent origin. There still is controversy and lack of adequate scientific data about the complete profile of risk-reduction interventions that are appropriate for people in developed countries as they pass through the latter third of the human life cycle. The size and health status of the older adult population is evolving at a rapid pace. It is, therefore, difficult to analyze all the variables so that we can understand the process and help guide it in constructive directions. Notwithstanding the complexity of the process, however, enough information is available to provide a reasonable scientific foundation for recommending a multidimensional health maintenance program. As new knowledge is acquired, the approach will be modified and made more comprehensive.

The task of implementing effective risk reduction requires a level of partnership and teamwork that is more complex and challenging than is usually encountered in the care of clinical illness. For the patient who feels ill, there is immediate motivation to do whatever is advised to regain a sense of well-being. In contrast, the person who feels relatively well must be motivated by the probability of future ill health and the possibility that doing something different now will be of benefit in the future. Present good health is not necessarily a strong motivator. Doubt about the certainty of future illness leaves room for questioning whether alteration of risk factors is necessary.

On the other side of the equation, physicians and other health professionals can all too readily adopt the same pattern of thinking. One's success in helping a group of elderly patients to avoid illness is difficult to quantify. The resolution of congestive heart failure, recovery from myocardial infarction or the setting and healing of a fracture are far more immediate sources of professional satisfaction and financial reward. Given these motivational disparities between curative and preventive medicine, the difficulties in elevating prevention to a mutually high priority are understandable.

The thesis underlying this chapter is that it is essential to accelerate our collective efforts to teach and practice cost-effective health promotion/disease prevention for the old as well as the young. In order to do this, there must be social commitment to allocate a larger fraction of public, private, and personal health care resources to prevention-oriented health and medical care. The goal must be to minimize the period of chronic illness and disability with its attendant high cost for the older population. A corollary need is to develop lower cost alternatives for the care of unavoidable illness that are consistent with the benefits that medical and nursing care can provide. The interrelated goals of health promotion and risk reduction in later life thus can be summarized in the following principles:

(1) Prevent or delay the onset of chronic disease and disability wherever possible.

(2) Reduce the severity of chronic diseases and disabilities that are not prevented.

(3) Maintain mental and physical health and functional independence as long as possible.

(4) Maximize the capacity to enjoy life in multiple dimensions as long as possible.

(5) Minimize discomfort and loss of independence and personal dignity during the terminal phase of life.

DEMOGRAPHIC TRENDS FAVORING INCREASED EMPHASIS ON HEALTH PROMOTION IN LATER LIFE

There has been a dramatic shift in patterns of disease causing death in the United States and other developed countries during the present century. The major killers in the early 1900s were the infections and contagious diseases. With the adoption of more hygienic community water supplies and sewage treatment; improved housing, working conditions, medical care, nutrition, and personal hygiene; and the advent of effective vaccines and antibiotics, chronic diseases have become the major causes of mortality in the latter half of the century.

Concurrent with the disease shift, there has been progressive lengthening of the average life expectancy in the United States from 45 years in 1900 to 75 years in the late 1980s. The increase in average life expectancy has resulted in unprecedented growth in the size and diversity of the over-60 population, with the most rapid growth in the over-85 age group. This trend is expected to accelerate as we move into the next century.

These health and demographic trends pose many problems for health and human service providers. The number of elderly persons requiring acute hospital, long-term, and home-care services continues to grow and will accelerate in the foreseeable future as the result of the demographic trends noted above. Thus it is essential that efforts accelerate to prepare for the challenges that lie ahead. Past methods of dealing with these issues from a social policy perspective already are proving to be grossly inadequate. Major shifts in a wide variety of areas will be necessary. The area most relevant to this discussion is the relative emphasis on preventive as opposed to curative and custodial care.

WHERE SHOULD DISEASE PREVENTION EFFORTS BE FOCUSED?

The three major diseases causing premature illness, disability, and death in the elderly generally are heart disease, cancer, and stroke. Heart disease, primarily coronary arteriosclerosis, heads the list with cancer and stroke second and third, respectively. It has been estimated that if all heart disease were eliminated there would be an increase of 16 years in average longevity compared to an average gain of 1.6 years if all cancers were eliminated (Beaver & Atkins, 1988). Thus, from the public health viewpoint, a high priority focus for disease prevention should continue to be on preventable forms of heart disease. The 30% reduction in the coronary heart disease death rate over the past two decades demonstrates that substantial progress has been made (Kannel & Vokonas, 1986). More substantial progress is possible as prevention-oriented life-style changes are more widely adopted. Cancer, the number two cause of death and chronic illness in the elderly, occurs in a variety of organ sites. Each site-specific cancer has its own unique profile of risk factors, many of which are still unknown. The most effective prevention-oriented efforts to date have been in the area of screening, early detection,

Table 2.1

Modifiable Risk Factors for Heart Disease and Stroke

Hypertension (primarily a risk factor for stroke)
Elevated LDL/low HDL cholesterol
Sedentary life-style
Smoking
Obesity > 20 percent above standard tables
Diabetes mellitus/hyperglycemia

and treatment of accessible anatomic sites such as breast, cervix, and skin. Dietary and environmental modification also are important for primary cancer prevention. More will be said about this later.

Stroke, the number three chronic disease killer in the elderly, primarily is due to atherosclerotic narrowing and occlusion of the arterial system of the brain. A small portion is due to hemorrhage and embolism (dislodged blood clots) of cerebral vessels. Hypertension is a major contributory cause of stroke and is amenable to medical therapy. Broader control of high blood pressure and other measures have reduced stroke mortality by 45% over the last 20 years and further progress is possible (Kannel & Vokonas, 1986).

There are a number of other acute and chronic illnesses to which the elderly are susceptible and for which effective preventive measures are available. These will be discussed in the next section.

RISK FACTORS THAT CAN BE MODIFIED IN LATER LIFE WITH BENEFICIAL RESULTS

Arteriosclerotic Heart Disease, Stroke, Peripheral Vascular Disease

The major modifiable risk factors for these conditions are listed in Table 2.1.

Hypertension

Chief among the modifiable risk factors is hypertension. Hypertension incidence increases with age and affects from 60% to 80% of people between the ages of 65 and 75 (Ostfeld, 1986). The trend continues on to older ages. It is estimated that uncontrolled high blood pressure accounts for 500,000 strokes and 1.5 million heart attacks per year. Persistent high blood pressure damages the walls of arteries causing the walls to become thicker and promotes the formation of plaques and clots inside the arteries. The beguiling characteristic of hypertension is its asymptomatic nature during the early stages when detection and therapy are most effective in preventing serious damage to the arteries, heart, brain, and kidneys. This fact argues strongly for expansion of blood pressure screening programs for older adults (Hypertension Detection and Followup Program Cooperative Group, 1979). In the elderly, systolic hypertension appears to be a more significant risk factor than diastolic hypertension. When present long enough to produce left ventricular hypertrophy, it is an even stronger predictor of coronary heart disease (Kannel, Gordon, & Offut, 1969).

The beneficial effects of lowering blood pressure have been demonstrated for older as well as middle-aged adults. For example, the European Working Party on Hypertension in the Elderly (1986) demonstrated an overall 38% to 58% reduction in cardiovascular deaths and a 60% reduction in morbidity in treated versus placebo groups between ages 60 and 79. Minimum benefit was demonstrated beyond age 79 (Amery et al., 1985; Amery et al., 1986).

Unhealthy Lipid Levels

There is a natural tendency for serum cholesterol levels to rise with increasing age in developed countries. It is widely recognized that blood lipid levels are important contributors to vascular disease of the heart, brain, and other organs. The primary etiologic mechanisms is the acceleration of cholesterol containing plaque development in the interior surface of arteries with progressive narrowing of the lumen. Complete occlusion leads to death of the cells whose blood supply is dependent upon the occluded artery.

The blood lipids that have been studied the longest with the largest data base are total cholesterol and triglycerides. Total cholesterol levels are statistically more powerful predictors of heart attacks and strokes than triglycerides. With advances in laboratory technology in recent decades, a variety of lipid fractions have been identified and their relationships to vascular disease studied.

Total cholesterol comprises several molecular fractions based upon the molecular weight of the associated lipoprotein molecule. High density lipoprotein (HDL) cholesterol has the largest molecular weight and plays a beneficial role in preventing or reducing the deposition of cholesterol in arterial plaques. Thus the higher the HDL cholesterol level in the blood, the lower the risk of arteriosclerotic disease. Low density lipoprotein (LDL) cholesterol has a lower molecular weight. High levels of LDL are associated with a higher risk of atherosclerotic disease, especially coronary disease. Very low density lipoprotein (VLDL) is the third and smallest of the major lipid fractions in the blood. It is composed mainly of triglyceride fatty acids coupled with lipoprotein.

As researchers have examined the relationships between various lipid fraction levels in the blood and the frequency of heart attacks over time, such as in the Framingham study, the ratio of LDL to HDL cholesterol has emerged as the strongest predictor. The higher the ratio, the greater the risk of heart attack. The risk increases rapidly above an LDL/HDL ratio of 3:1 (Smith, Karmally, & Brown, 1987). Conversely, a program designed to reduce the ratio, including diet, exercise, medication, and abstinence from smoking, has potential to reduce the risk of heart attack in the elderly (National Cholesterol Eduction Program Expert Panel, 1988). The LDL fraction is the major fraction of total cholesterol. When total cholesterol goes up or down, the LDL fraction typically is the one most involved.

Although some studies suggest elevated cholesterol is a less significant risk factor for the aged (Kaiser & Morley, 1990), recent consensus guidelines emphasize cholesterol goal levels of 200 mg/dl or less for total cholesterol, 130 mg/dl or less for LDL cholesterol, and 45 mg/dl or higher for HDL cholesterol. Dietary guidelines to achieve healthier lipid levels are to maintain fat intake at no more than 30% of average daily calories and an unsaturated/saturated fat ratio of 2:1. Unsaturated fats should be equally divided between monounsaturated and polyunsaturated fatty acids (National Cholesterol Education Program Expert Panel, 1988). Largely eliminating animal fat from the diet and using fish and skinned poultry as the sources of dietary protein help accomplish this goal. Limiting refined sugar and including high fiber foods (vegetables, fruits, whole grain bread, oat bran, and so forth) also contribute to maintaining healthier lipid levels.

Sedentary Life-Style

There is a general tendency for people to "slow down" as they age due to a variety of factors. These include physiologic aging changes with partial loss of the youthful energy reservoir and a social expectation in contemporary society that one should slow down with age. There also has been a major shift in physical work demands as we have moved from a manual-labor-oriented, agricultural, predominantly rural society to a largely mechanized, urbanized, automation-oriented culture. Most people must make a disciplined effort to get aerobic exercise today, whereas a century ago strenuous physical work was a necessary part of everyday life from childhood to old age for most people.

Lack of aerobic physical exercise is a broadly significant risk factor for heart disease and a variety of other health problems including obesity, osteoporosis, glucose intolerance, and skeletal muscle atrophy. Conversely, maintenance of a regular pattern of physical activity that stimulates the body's aerobic metabolism has been called "the closest thing we have to an anti-aging pill" (Leaf, 1973).

A number of studies over the past two decades have demonstrated the beneficial health effects of regular physical exercise in modest proportions for middle-aged and older adults (Paffenbarger, Wang, & Hyde, 1978; Shepard, 1990). The earlier the exercise habit is established, the greater the health benefits. A controlled study on younger adults has demonstrated the many potential lifelong benefits of different levels of exercise. A study of Harvard alumni by Paffenbarger, Wang, and Hyde (1986) showed that people who typically walked 5 to 10 miles per week reduced their mortality rate by 10% as compared to sedentary people. Those who walked 20 to 25 miles per week experienced a 40% lower death rate. As expected, most of the reduced mortality was due to a lower heart attack rate.

A widely accepted physiologic criterion for maintenance of aerobic physical fitness is work, recreation, or an exercise routine that will stimulate the heart to beat at 70% of the theoretic maximum achievable heart rate for at least 20 minutes, at least three times a week. A general formula for calculating the theoretic maximum heart rate is 220 minus age for males, and 225 minus age for females. For example, the calculation for a 65-year-old woman would be $225 - 65 = 160 \times .70 = 112$ beats/minute as the target pulse rate during exercise. Individualized adjustments need to be made for health status, medications, and other factors. Older adults who are not accustomed to regular aerobic activity should work into a program gradually under the guidance of their personal physician.

Smoking

There are no demonstrable health benefits from smoking at any age. All health effects are negative. The list of mechanisms by which physiologic function is impaired and the pathophysiologic soil for disease is fertilized by chronic smoking grows longer with each passing year. Chief among these is the overpowering evidence that chronic smoking is a major risk factor for atherosclerosis, particularly heart attacks and peripheral vascular disease (Ostfeld, 1986; U.S. Department of Health and Human Services, 1983). The strong association between chronic cigarette smoking and lung cancer, pulmonary emphysema, cancer of the esophagus, larynx, oral cavity, lip, and bladder is also well documented (Fielding, 1985; Mattson, Pollack, & Cullen, 1987; U.S. Department of Health, Education and Welfare, 1979). The contribution of chronic smoking to osteoporosis, digestive disorders, altered drug metabolism and nutrient bioavailability are less dramatic, but nevertheless significant, negative health effects.

The research literature does not yet contain strong evidence that smoking cessation after age 65 measurably reduces the vascular disease death rate. There are wide individual differences in susceptibility to the variety of negative health effects of smoking, including risk of heart attacks. It may be that those most susceptible to accelerated coronary atherosclerosis from smoking have died prior to age 65. Another possibility is that there is diminished ability of the elderly person's arterial system to benefit from smoking cessation after age 65, and longer follow-up periods are necessary to demonstrate differences in death rates. It also should be recognized that other confounding, nonreversible negative health effects of lifelong smoking on longevity obscures whatever gains may be present from smoking cessation.

From the standpoint of disease prevention, however, it is prudent to extrapolate what is known from the many larger scale studies of younger adults (i.e., smoking is harmful to an aging body with deteriorating cardiac, pulmonary, gastrointestinal, genitourinary and other functions). Every effort should be made to persuade and assist the elderly smoker to quit.

Obesity

Life insurance company mortality data and other studies have repeatedly demonstrated the negative health effects of obesity. From the standpoint of clinical care, obesity is a common coexisting health problem with hypertension, diabetes mellitus, degenerative arthritis, and a number of other health problems. For some people, even modest reduction in body weight enhances the ability to control blood pressure and blood glucose levels, and for some this is the only treatment required. Hypertension and diabetes, often accompanied by unhealthy lipid levels are, of course, important risk factors for arteriosclerotic vascular disease.

Obesity in an elderly adult is often part of a vicious web of health problems and risk factors. Being overweight makes physical activity less attractive and often painful because of accelerated degeneration of the weight-bearing joints of the legs (especially knees and hips). A larger percentage of ingested calories are converted to fat in the presence of a sedentary activity pattern. The perfusion demands of excess fat place unhealthy demands on the heart and circulatory system. Respiratory function is restricted because of crowding of the diaphragm and the increased work of respiration. Oxygenation of the blood in the lungs may be reduced, thus compromising full oxygenation of peripheral tissues. Obese skin folds trap moisture and proteinaceous secretions and breakdown products, thus increasing the risk of local fungal and bacterial infections. The list goes on and on.

Modifying the habits of an elderly person who has experienced lifelong obesity is a challenging task. For people who have reached their late seventies and older in this state, the gains in reduced morbidity and length of life from weight reduction efforts may be minimal. Further, if individuals cannot be easily motivated to modify their diet and increase daily physical activity, intervention is not worth pursuing. From the standpoint of prevention programming, the target group for weight control should be people in their fifties, sixties, and early seventies who are still able to be active and who can be educated and motivated to begin a long-term weight reduction and weight control program.

In considering obesity as a risk factor, one must also recognize that, for some people, genetically determined longevity factors may be more important determinants of length of life and health than the risk factors under control of the individual. Thus enthusiasm for intervention must be tempered by the wisdom that comes from recognizing the larger picture.

A recommended weight range for older adults is to be within plus or minus 15% of the weights listed in standard Metropolitan Life weight tables (Metropolitan Life Insurance Co., 1983). Development of separate height/weight tables for people over 65 has been proposed but has not been widely accepted as clinically useful. However, it has been noted that modest rise in body mass indices is statistically associated with lower age-related mortality (Andres, 1985).

Diabetes Mellitus

The prevalence of diabetes and glucose intolerance increases rapidly in older adults and also is positively correlated with obesity (U.S. Department of Health and Human Services, 1988). There is substantial epidemiologic evidence to suggest that the prevalence of adult onset, non-insulin-dependent diabetes in adults could be measurably reduced in developed countries if lifelong nutrition and physical activity patterns were modified (Hess, 1983). The dietary recommendation in the Surgeon General's Report on Nutrition and Health for persons who have already developed diabetes (high fiber-complex CHO/low refined sugar, low saturated fat) approach the diets consumed in primitive societies where the incidence of diabetes is low. If all adults followed this type of diet and exercised regularly, it is likely that the prevalence of diabetes in older adults gradually would diminish in the decades ahead.

The modifications suggested by available data include:

(1) Reduction in refined sugar consumption to well below 75 pounds per year. The current average U.S. consumption is around 127 pounds per year (U.S. Department of Health and Human Services, 1988).

(2) Adoption of a diet with a high proportion of complex carbohydrates to approximately 50% of total calories. The current U.S. average is 22% (Garrison & Somer, 1985).

(3) A consistent pattern of physical activity that would maintain aerobic metabolism and body weight at health levels, as suggested earlier.

(4) Maintenance of adequate chromium nutrition. There is a growing body of evidence demonstrating the importance of chromium and other nutrients in the control of glucose metabolism (Urberg & Zemel, 1987).

Osteopenia (Osteoporosis/Osteomalacia)

Osteopenia is the term applied to demineralization of bone. It is the underlying cause for most bone fractures and spinal deformities in the elderly. There are multiple risk factors for osteopenia. The loss of estrogen production at the time of the female menopause is a well-established risk factor. In addition to hormone deficiencies, genetic background, physical inactivity, medications (i.e., corticosteroid, theophylline, and others); high alcohol and caffeine intake; nutritional factors such as inadequate vitamin D, high acid ash diet (i.e., high protein, deficient trace elements), and smoking are risk factors.

The fact that appearance of clinically evident osteopenia correlates so highly with the postmenopausal state in women and is relatively rare in elderly men who do not experience a comparable sex hormone reduction argues strongly for the role of hormone deficiency as a risk factor for osteoporosis. This hypothesis is further supported by the effectiveness of estrogen replacement therapy reducing the frequency, progress, and severity of osteoporosis in postmenopausal women (Bellantoni & Blackman, 1988).

The use of estrogen alone to retard bone demineralization was associated with an increased incidence of endometrial cancer. The more recent, more physiologic protocol of cycled estrogen and progesterone replacement therapy has essentially eliminated the endometrial cancer concern and appears to improve the prognosis for women who develop breast cancer (Hammond, Jelousek, Creasman, & Parker, 1979). Estrogen is usually recommended at the time of, or within five years of, menopause in order to slow postmenopausal bone demineralization (Heidrich & Thompson, 1987). It is not as yet clear, however, how long cycled estrogen/progesterone replacement therapy should be continued. As yet there is no strong evidence against continuing hormone replacement into the seventies and eighties, particularly in women otherwise at high risk for osteoporosis. Nutritional factors can influence the development of osteoporosis. Calcium supplementation sometimes is suggested, but the role of calcium intake in maintaining bone density is controversial. Calcium nutrition is, however, considered important enough in the elderly that a recommended daily allowance (RDA) for calcium of 1,000 to 1,500 mg/day for post menopausal women has been proposed (Schneider, Vining, Hadley, & Farnham, 1986).

Cancers

A number of cancers in older adults are amenable to secondary prevention, that is, early detection and treatment. These include cancer of the breast, cervix, uterus, skin, rectum, colon, and prostate.

Breast Cancer

Breast cancer incidence is greatest in women over the age of 50 (Gambrell, 1988). In general, breast cancers diagnosed and treated in stages I and II (in-site or local spread only) have substantially better cure and survival rates than cancers detected in stages III and IV (regional and generalized spread). The least expensive method of screening for breast cancer is breast self-examination (BSE) on a regularly monthly or weekly basis. The friction free (soap suds, oil on the skin) method is the most sensitive. Every woman should be taught and encouraged to regularly perform BSE throughout adult life. BSE is especially important from age 50 onward. Suspicious areas should immediately be brought to a physician's attention.

Mammography is the most sensitive method for breast cancer screening. It will detect suspicious lesions long before they can be felt by the woman or her physician. All suspicious lesions should be biopsied. The American Cancer Society recommends annual mammograms for all women over 50 (Gambrell, 1988). The U.S. Preventive Services Task Force recommends mammograms every one to two years and discontinuance at age 74, if results are consistently negative (Woolf, Kamerow, Lawrence, Medalie, & Estes, 1990).

Cervical Cancer

Cervical cancer is readily detected by pelvic exam and Papanicolaou (Pap) smear. Early lesions can be cured simply and inexpensively by local excision, freezing, cautery, or laser therapy. More advanced lesions require more extensive surgery and radiation and/or chemotherapy. the difference in cost, pain, and suffering is enormous.

Most women in the current sixty-plus age group are not accustomed to having regular Pap smears (Celentano, 1988). This is due in part to the misconception that after menopause Pap smears no longer are necessary. As a consequence, in older women cervical cancers typically are further advanced at the time of diagnosis than is true for younger women. The use of estrogen in postmenopausal women may extend the "at risk" period for cervical cancer, so yearly Pap smears should be recommended for women over 60. After three negative tests, screening may be discontinued at the physician's discretion (Butler, 1988).

Uterine Cancer

Uterine cancer should be suspected in any postmenopausal woman who notes vaginal bleeding, unless she is on cyclic hormone replacement therapy. In the latter case, midcycle vaginal bleeding should be regarded as an early warning symptom. Early diagnosis and treatment usually results in a cure.

Cancers of the Skin and Oropharynx

Cancers of the skin and oropharynx also are accessible to early diagnosis and cure. A lump that persists or a sore that does not heal should be promptly brought to a physician's attention for diagnosis and care.

Cancer of the Rectum and Colon

Cancer of the rectum and colon can be easily diagnosed and, if found early, cured. Bowel cancers typically begin as polyps that can be removed through a scope. Blood in the stool is the most common early warning symptom of colorectal polyps and cancer. Annual testing of three stool samples for occult blood is recommended by the American Cancer Society for all people over age 50. Sigmoidoscope annually for two years and, if negative, every three to five years thereafter is recommended after age 50. Epidemiologic data have been developed that show the high-fiber diet consumed in underdeveloped countries is associated with a substantially lower incidence of colorectal cancer than the low-fiber diet of developed countries (Burkitt, Walker, & Painter, 1972; Greenwald, Lanza, & Eddy, 1987). Whether high fiber alone is the major dependent variable remains to be seen. However, recent research shows that a high-fiber diet shortens fecal transit time and reduces exposure of bowel mucosa to ammonia-producing bacteria (Clinton, Bostwick, Olson, Mangram, & Visek, 1988).

Even though all the answers are not in, it is probably prudent to recommend a dietary fiber intake in the range of 25 to 35 grams a day beginning as early in life as possible. Most older adults will need to use fiber supplements to achieve this level and avoid gaining weight. Oat bran and psyllium hydrophilic mycelioid are recommended as the primary fiber supplement sources because of their greater effect on cholesterol reduction and lower phytase content than wheat bran.

Prostatic Cancer

Prostatic cancer is the second most common cancer in elderly men and is twice as common in black men than in white men (Huben & Murphy, 1986). The risk factors for prostate cancer are not well defined though some nutritional factors have been suspected.

Current screening techniques for prostatic cancer are not very effective in detecting early lesions. The early cancers typically are discovered incidentally as the result of surgery for the more common tumor, benign prostatic hypertrophy (BPH). Both BPH and chronic prostatitis can obscure a growing carcinoma. However, since the posterior prostate is accessible to palpation via rectal examination, older men should have an annual rectal/prostate examination.

Infection

Immunization against two potentially fatal infections in the elderly—influenza A and B and pneumococcal pneumonia—are effective risk-reduction strategies. The impaired defense system against infection present in many older adults makes them more susceptible to infectious disease.

Influenza

Influenza (flu) vaccines are reformulated each year based on epidemiologic tracking of the prevalent strains during the early phase of the annual flu season. Vaccines are prepared accordingly and are ready for administration in late September or early October each year. People over 65 should be encouraged to receive flu vaccine annually (Morbidity and Mortality Weekly Report, 1988). Contrary to what most lay people think, flu vaccine does not protect against the myriad gastrointestinal and respiratory viruses that afflict old and young every winter and spring.

Pneumonia

Pneumococcal vaccine protects against infection by the bacterium streptococcus (formerly pneumococcus) pneumonia. It is prepared from a capsular antigen. One immunization is recommended for people 65 or older (Immunization Practices Advisory Committee, 1984). Its major benefit is protection against pneumococcal pneumonia, a relatively mild, easily treatable condition in young people but a serious and sometimes fatal disease in the elderly.

Tetanus

Tetanus immunization every 10 years is required to maintain immunity in adults (Advisory Committee on Immunization Practices, 1985). The same schedule is recommended for older adults but the intervals may be shortened as more is learned about the stability of immunity in older people. Active elderly who are at risk for penetrating trauma is the group for whom tetanus immunization is most important.

Nutrient Deficiencies and Disturbances of Nutrient Bioavailability

Calories in the diet provide the energy substrates that fuel the body's metabolic machinery, much like coal, gas, oil, and wood are used as energy sources for man-made machinery. On the other hand, nutrients in the diet provide the molecular building blocks that the body uses to construct and maintain its marvelously complex anatomic and biochemical machinery. An ongoing balance of both calories and nutrients in the diet is essential for optimum health.

The key issue in nutrition management and its relationship to long-term health is balance. Too much or too little of any of the broad array of nutrients and caloric sources that are part of a well-balanced diet can, over time, be harmful. The human organism has a remarkable capacity to adapt to a wide variety of excesses and deficiencies on a short-term basis. However, over prolonged periods, deficiencies of calories and essential individual nutrients lead to severe malfunctioning. Vitamin and mineral deficiencies lead to development of many diseases. Nutritional deficiencies in older adults also set the stage for disease development or chronic disability. Impairment of wound healing is one example of a nutritional deficit disorder.

The issue of nutrient bioavailability is of greater concern in older as compared to young adults. The quantity of nutrient ingested is only one part of the nutritional balance equation. Other considerations are the amount digested and absorbed, the amount available and usable at key metabolic sites, and the amount excreted in urine, feces, and sweat. As people age, there is a tendency for the digestive/absorption process to be less efficient (less gastric acid, pepsin secretion, and so forth); drugs and fiber may form complexes with and prevent absorption of some nutrients; and the absorptive surface and efficiency of the bowel tends to diminish with age. Some drugs, such as diuretics, promote increased excretion of some nutrients in addition to sodium (e.g., K, Mg, Ca, Zn); other drugs may compete with essential nutrients at cellular metabolic sites (e.g., INH/pyridoxine; phenytoin/folic acid; folate antagonists/folate).

The combined effects of marginal nutrient intake, suboptional digestion/absorption, impaired utilization, and altered excretion in an older person may produce metabolically significant impairment of several physiologic functions. If continued, the nutrient deficiencies can lead to onset or worsening of clinically apparent disease. The underlying culprit (nutrient deficiency) typically goes unrecognized by clinical care givers. By then, irreversible pathologic damage may be present. The optimum period for effective prevention is long since past.

The prevention-oriented message to be derived from the above is that, from the standpoint of clinical care, older adults consuming 1,500 to 1,800 calories per day or fewer (which is average for most elderly) should be advised to take a daily 100% RDA level vitamin/mineral/trace element supplement as part of their "health insurance" program (Nutrition Action Health Letter, 1988). This level of nutrient supplementation is safe, balanced, and nontoxic. It safely adds to the often marginal intake of many nutrients in the daily diet and helps to compensate for the kinds of bioavailability problems discussed above that are clinically unrecognized.

On the other hand, the use of megadoses (several times the RDA) of single or multiple nutrient supplements is to be *strongly discouraged* unless specifically prescribed by a knowledgeable physician for a specific purpose. Megadose vitamins and minerals are potentially toxic and cause imbalance in the dynamics of other nutrients (Alfin-Slater, 1988; Rudman & Williams, 1983).

Accident Prevention

Accidental death rates for people over 65 are double that for younger people. Most accidents are preventable by more careful attention to the home or to vehicle safety. This action can prevent falls and unnecessary fractures.

The evidence that routine use of vehicle seat belts lessens severity of injury and saves lives is well documented and has been translated into law in many states (Goldbaum, Remington, Powell, Hoglin, & Gentry, 1986). Older people are more likely to sustain fractures, have slower recovery from injury, and often have more prolonged disability than younger people. Thus routine seat belt use should be actively encouraged for older adults.

PRACTICAL ISSUES IN EDUCATING
OLDER PEOPLE TO ADOPT
HEALTHIER LIFE-STYLES

Health promotion/disease prevention requires a partnership between health professionals and their patients/clients. The professional has the knowledge and technical skills to assist with the implementation of appropriate screening and intervention procedures. These can reduce the probability of premature illness, disability, and death. The task is relatively quick, simple, inexpensive, and passive for the patient/client for procedures such as blood sampling, blood pressure measurement, immunization, mammography, and glaucoma screening. On the other hand, the professional can recommend and educate but is relatively limited when the patient/client must assume active responsibility for implementing dietary modifications, an accelerated exercise program, smoking cessation, weight reduction, seat belt use, or improved dental hygiene.

Many older people are more enthusiastic, more motivated, and have more time for pursuing health promoting activities than younger people. They no longer take good health for granted as they see many of their peers, relatives, and friends succumbing to chronic, incurable illness and finally death. Many feel that they would do anything to avoid prolonged disability. They want to retain the capacity to live an active, meaningful life as long as possible, and when that period is over, "come quickly sweet death."

Other oldsters take a more fatalistic attitude. "What's done is done." "It's too late to change now." "My Aunt Phoebe smoked and chewed tobacco until she was 91, and it didn't seem to hurt her. I'll take my chances the way I am." The expressions of apathy and fatalism take many forms and are part of the larger reality that must be faced. All of this serves to underscore the point that personal interest and motivation toward future health status is probably *the* major individual determinant of successful involvement in a health promotion program.

Other practical issues that must be addressed on an individual basis include the following:

- *Mental, emotional functional status.* Is the person capable of sustained involvement in a program that requires continuing, disciplined, goal-oriented thought and behavior?
- *Current physical capabilities.* What is the level of functional independence? What physical limitations need to be taken into account?

- *Life-style and attitudes of close significant others.* To what extent do the life-style and attitudes of close significant others influence the behavior, attitudes, and ability of the person to change?
- *Nutrition decisions.* Who prepares the food and who makes the important nutrition decisions?
- *Budget decisions.* What is the size and flexibility of the person's discretionary budget? How does this influence the ability to improve nutrition, increase physical fitness activities, and obtain professional and institutionally based prevention-oriented services?
- *Other factors.* What are the strengths and liabilities of the individual's socioeconomic, occupational, cultural, and educational background? What opportunities and limitations do these factors create?

The geriatric population is extremely heterogenous on each of the issues raised. The practical implication is the necessity of individualization and flexibility of programming. Health maintenance programs are thus more difficult organizationally and potentially more costly for this age group than for younger people. Yet, the yield in quality months of life gained and dollars saved for hospital and nursing home care may be substantial (Shin, 1983).

In pursuing health promotion among the elderly, it is essential to remember that much remains to be learned about which prevention-oriented procedures are effective when initiated in the latter 20 to 30 years of the human life cycle. The old adage "the sooner, the better," is certainly applicable to most elements of prevention-oriented care.

The main question being raised here, however, is, "How late is too late?" The answer in many areas is that no one as yet knows and opinion is divided. A few of the issues that fall into this category include the following:

- Does increasing calcium and vitamin intake late in life retard the progression of osteoporosis?
- Does increasing dietary fiber content late in life reduce the incidence of polyps and cancer of the bowel?
- Does reducing sodium and increasing potassium, calcium, or magnesium in the diet defer or prevent the development of hypertension in some people?
- Will improved trace element nutrition (zinc, copper, silicon, selenium, chromium) substantially reduce the prevalence of impaired cellular immunity, glucose intolerance, dark adaptation, taste acuity, unhealthy lipids, osteoporosis, and other physiologic impairments commonly seen in the elderly?

Humanitarian, self-interest, and cost-containment considerations demand that we press on in our efforts to further refine and demonstrate the value of

health-promoting, risk-reducing procedures and activities for the latter years
of human life.

REFERENCES

Advisory Committee on Immunization Practices. (1985). Leads from MMWR—Diphtheria,
  tetanus and pertussis: Guidelines for vaccine prophylaxis and other preventive measures.
  Journal of the American Medical Association, 254, 895-900.
Alfin-Slater, R. B. (1988). Vitamin use and abuse in the elderly. In J. E. Morley (Moderator),
  Nutrition in the elderly. *Annals of Internal Medicine, 109,* 890-904.
Amery, A., Birkenhager, W., Brixko, R., Bulpitt, C., Clement, D., Deruyttere, M.,
  DeShaepdryver, A., Dollery, C., Fagard, R., Forette, F., & associates. (1985). Mortality and
  morbidity results from the European working party on high blood pressure in the elderly
  trial. *Lancet, 1,* 349-354.
Amery, A., Birkenhager, W., Brixko, R., Bulpitt, C., Clement, D., Deruyttere, M.,
  DeSchaepdryver, A., Dollery, C., Fagard, R., Forette, F., & associates. (1986). Efficacy of
  antihypertensive drug treatment according to age, sex, blood pressure and previous cardio-
  vascular disease in patients over the age of 60. *Lancet, 2,* 589-592.
Andres, R. (1985). Mortality and obesity: The rational for age-specific height-weight tables. In
  R. Andres, E. L. Bierman, & W. R. Hazzard (Eds.), *Principles of geriatric medicine.* New
  York: McGraw-Hill.
Beaver, T., & Atkins, D. (1988). Cardiovascular risk factors in the elderly: Is intervention really
  necessary? *Clinical Report on Aging, 2,* 1-19.
Bellantoni, M. F., & Blackman, M. R. (1988). Osteoporosis: Diagnostic screening and its place
  in current care. *Geriatrics, 43,* 63-70.
Burkitt, D. P., Walker, A. R. P., Painter, N. S. (1972). Effect of dietary fiber on stools, transit
  times and its role in the causation of disease. *Lancet, 2,* 1408-1410.
Butler, R. N. (1988). Pap smears for cervical cancer: Don't neglect the elderly. *Geriatrics, 43,*
  13-16.
Celentano, D. D. (1988). Updated approach to screening for cervical cancer in older women.
  Geriatrics, 43, 37-48.
European Working Party on Hypertension in the Elderly. (1986). Statement on hypertension in
  the elderly. *Journal of the American Medical Association, 256,* 70-74.
Fielding, J. E. (1985). Smoking: Health effects and control. *New England Journal of Medicine,
  313,* 491-498.
Gambrell, R. D. (1988). Cancer in the older woman: Diagnosis and prevention. *Geriatrics, 43,*
  27-36.
Garrison, R. H., & Somer, E. (1985). *The nutrition desk reference.* New Canaan, CT: Keats.
Goldbaum, G. M., Remington, P. L., Powell, K. E., Hoglin, G. C., & Gentry, E. M. (1986). The
  behavioral risk factors survey group. Failure to use seat belts in the United States: The
  1981-83 behavioral risk factor surveys. *Journal of the American Medical Association, 87,*
  1178-1188.
Gruchow, H. W., Anderson, A. D., Barbonick, I. J., & Sobocenski, K. A. (1988). Postmenopausal
  use of estrogen and occlusion of coronary arteries. *American Heart Journal, 115,* 954-962.
Greenwald, P., Lanza, E., Eddy, G. A. (1987). Dietary fiber in the reduction of colon cancer risk.
  Journal of the American Dietetic Association, 87, 1178-1188.

Hammond, C. B., Jelousek, F. R., Creasman, W. T., & Parker, R. T. (1979). Effects of long-term estrogen replacement therapy on neoplasia. *American Journal of Obstetrics and Gynecology, 133*, 537-547.

Hess, J. W. (1983). Obesity and diabetes in the context of disease prevention/health promotion. In J. W. Hess, M. R. Liepman, & T. J. Ruane (Eds.), *Family practice and preventive medicine.* New York: Human Sciences Press.

Huben, R. P., & Murphy, G. P. (1986). Prostate cancer: An update. *CA—A Cancer Journal for Clinicians, 36*, 274-292.

Hypertension Detection and Follow-up Program Cooperative Group. (1979). Five year findings in the hypertension detection and follow-up program II: Mortality by race, sex and age. *Journal of the American Medical Association, 242*, 2572-2577.

Immunization Practices Advisory Committee. (1984). Pneumococcal polysaccharide vaccine usage—United States. *Annals of Internal Medicine, 111*, 348-350.

Kannel, W. B., Gordon, T., & Offut, D. (1969). Left ventricular hypertrophy by electrocardiogram: Prevalence, incidence, and mortality in the Framingham study. *Annals of Internal Medicine, 71*, 89-105.

Kannel, W. B., & Vokonas, P. S. (1986). Primary risk factors for coronary heart disease in the elderly: The Framingham study. In N. K. Wenger, C. D. Furberg, & E. Pitt (Eds.), *Coronary heart disease in the elderly.* New York: Elsevier.

Leaf, A. (1973, October). Unusual longevity: The common denominators. *Hospital Practice, 8*, 68-75.

MacMahon, S. W., Cutler, J. A., Furberg, C. D., & Payne, G. H. (1986). The effects of drug treatment for hypertension on morbidity and mortality from cardiovascular disease: A review of randomized controlled trials progress. *Cardiovascular Diseases, 29*(1), 99-118.

Mattson, M. E., Pollack, E. S., & Cullen, J. W. (1987). What are the odds that smoking will kill you? *American Journal of Public Health, 77*, 425-431.

Metropolitan Life Insurance Company. (1983). Metropolitan height and weight tables. *Statistical Bulletin, 64*, 2-9.

Morbidity and Mortality Weekly. (1988). *37*(23). (6/17/88).

Nutrition Action Health Letter. (1988). 15.

National Cholesterol Education Program Expert Panel. (1988). Report of the national cholesterol education program expert panel on detection, evaluation and treatment of high blood cholesterol in adults. *Archives of Internal Medicine, 148*, 36-69.

Ostfeld, A. M. (1986). The potential for primary prevention of coronary heart disease in the elderly. In N. K. Wenger, C. D. Furberg, & E. Pitt (Eds.), *Coronary heart disease in the elderly.* New York: Elsevier.

Paffenbarger, R. S., Wang, A. L., & Hyde, R. T. (1978). Physical activity as an index of heart attack risk in college alumni. *American Journal of Epidemiology, 108*, 161-175.

Paffenbarger, R. S., Wang, A. L., & Hyde, R. T. (1986). Physical activity, all cause mortality and longevity of college alumni. *New England Journal of Medicine, 314*, 605-613.

Rudman, D., & Williams, P. J. (1983). Megadose vitamins: Use and misuse. *New England Journal of Medicine, 309*, 488-489.

Schneider, E. L., Vining, E. M., Hadley, E. C., & Farnham, B. A. (1986). Recommended dietary allowances in the elderly. *New England Journal of Medicine, 314*, 157-160.

Shin, D. H. (1983). Prevention of blindness and preservation of vision as part of primary care. In J. W. Hess, M. R. Liepman, & T. J. Ruane (Eds.), *Family practice and preventive medicine* (pp. 388-406). New York: Human Services Press.

Smith, D. A., Karmally, W., & Brown, V. (1987). Treating hyperlipidemia: Part I—Whether and when in the elderly. *Geriatrics, 42*, 33-44.

Tinetti, M. E., Speechley, M., & Ginter, S. F. (1988). Risk factors for falls among elderly persons living in the community. *New England Journal of Medicine, 319*, 1701-1707.

Urberg, M., & Zemel, M. B. (1987). Evidence for synergism between chromium and nicontinic acide in the control of glucose tolerance in elderly humans. *Metabolism, 36*, 866-869.

U.S. Department of Health and Human Services. (1983). *The health consequences of smoking: Cardiovascular disease. A report of the surgeon general* (DHHS Publication No. PHS 84-50204). Washington, DC: Government Printing Office.

U.S. Department of Health and Human Services. (1988). *Surgeon general's report on nutrition and health* (DHHS Publication No. 88-50210). Washington, DC: Government Printing Office.

U.S. Department of Health, Education and Welfare. (1979). *Smoking and health: A report of the surgeon general* (DHEW Publication No. PHS 79-50066). Washington, DC: Government Printing Office.

Woolf, S. H., & Kamerow, D. B., Lawrence, R. S., Medalie, J. H., & Estes, E. H. (1990). The periodic health examination of older adults: The recommendations of the U.S. Preventive Services Task Force. *Journal of the American Geriatrics Society, 38*, 933-942.

Chapter 3

DRUG USE AND MISUSE AMONG THE ELDERLY

MARTHA J. MILLER

MEDICATION USE

The focus on the aging of America in recent decades has prompted a plea for increased understanding of medication use and the factors that influence drug therapy in the elderly. Currently, the elderly represent approximately 11.5% of the population in the United States, but this relatively small group accounts for 25% to 30% of the country's drug expenditures. By comparison, the elderly consume more medications than any other age group.

The actual use of prescribed medications in the elderly is difficult to interpret. Studies report the average medication consumption based on both new and refill prescriptions. According to a report by Kasper (1982), the average noninstitutionalized older person filled more than 10 prescriptions (new and refill) per year. Many of these prescriptions are for antianxiety agents and hypnotics. Due to the prevalence of chronic disease among the elderly, however, most prescriptions are for analgesics and cardiovascular preparations. This information demonstrates that prescription drug use is a rule rather than an exception in the elderly.

In addition to prescription medications, the elderly routinely take nonprescription (over-the-counter or OTC) drugs. Estimates in the literature vary, but several authors indicate the overwhelming majority of elderly patients routinely take nonprescription medications. The apparently common use of OTC drugs is supported by the fact that nearly one third of all medication expenditures by the elderly is for nonprescription drugs. Many elderly must pay for medications out of their own pockets. Since nonprescription drugs are generally less expensive than prescription drugs, the popularity of OTC medications with the elderly is not surprising.

Projections for the turn of the century estimate that the percentage of the elderly in the U.S. population will double. It is assumed similar patterns of disease management will prevail, and thus an increasing amount of medications will be consumed by the elderly.

The past, present, and future use of drugs in the elderly has been, and will be, accompanied by medication-related problems. Both patients and health care providers contribute to these problems. An awareness of some of the risks associated with medicating the elderly is important for all health care practitioners.

DISRUPTION OF RATIONAL DRUG USE IN THE ELDERLY

Several factors can contribute to the possibility of medication use problems and the disruption of rational therapy in the elderly. These factors include intentional and unintentional medication misuse, adverse drug reactions, lack of appreciation of the effects of aging, and inaccurate medical diagnosis. Some of these factors are linked to the patient, while others are attributed to health care professionals.

Medication Misuse or Noncompliance

Noncompliance can be defined as the failure of patients to follow instructions provided regarding the use of medication. This definition suggests noncompliance is more than a failure to take a dose of medication. Noncompliance encompasses failure to have a prescription filled, premature discontinuation of treatment, excessive medication consumption, and other misuse issues. The impact of noncompliance can be very significant in the elderly.

There is a persistent misconception that the elderly have a higher rate of noncompliance than younger patients. Reexamination of earlier literature indicates the rate of compliance in the elderly is similar to that in patients of all age groups. There may, however, be different reasons for noncompliance among patients of different ages.

A broad viewpoint of medication misuse departs from assuming patients who do not take their medications as prescribed have no rational basis for their noncompliance. To the contrary, most elderly patients often have sound reasons for not using their medications as directed. Perhaps one of these reasons with the most impact is medication cost. At times, medication cost is the reason people fail to have a prescription filled. It is important to note that 20% of the elderly's out-of-pocket (nonreimbursed) health expenditures are for medications. Many older individuals selectively take their medications on the basis of perceived importance (e.g., "heart medication") and the cost of the prescription. Another important consideration of medication misuse and the elderly is the possibility of failure to understand the proper dosage or times to take a particular drug. When therapy becomes more complicated (i.e., the number of medications to take increases), it is possible that a misunderstanding could take place. The prescriber must be sensitive to this information and willing to consider cost and take additional time to ensure the medication directions are clear and understood.

Adverse Drug Reactions

Adverse reactions to drugs comprise a significant problem in the care of the elderly. An adverse drug reaction can be defined as an unintended, untoward, harmful, or noxious response to a drug occurring at dosage levels used in humans for disease prevention, diagnosis, or therapy. The actual incidence of adverse drug reactions (ADRs) in the elderly is uncertain. Discrepancies in these data are due in part to differences in study populations, methods used to detect unwanted effects, and the definition of an adverse drug reaction. Recent reassessment, however, shows at least 10% of elderly admitted to hospitals are admitted secondary to an adverse drug reaction. Hospital staff are familiar with admissions of older persons for suspected ADRs. Many drugs are implicated, but a few bear mentioning due to their high use among the elderly and their potential to cause toxicity.

As previously noted, cardiovascular (heart and circulation) drugs frequently are prescribed for elderly patients. Into this category falls digoxin, diuretics, and antihypertensives. Digoxin is used to treat heart failure, diuretics are used to remove fluid from the body, and antihypertensive medications are used to treat high blood pressure. Digoxin often is implicated in drug-induced hospitalizations because of its inherent toxicity and frequency of use. Diuretics can lead to dehydration and electrolyte (salt) disturbances. Overly aggressive treatment with antihypertensives can result in postural, or positional, drops in blood pressure, fainting, or even a fall. Of course, other drugs can be associated with adverse effects. In general, medications that can cause ADRs are those prescribed most frequently without proper consideration of drug pharmacology and aging physiology.

Any number of reasons for the occurrence of ADRs in the elderly has been suggested. Attempts have been made to profile the older individual at risk for an adverse drug experience. Perhaps the best attempt to identify risk factors predisposing the elderly to adverse reactions is outlined by Michocki and Lamy (1988). They developed the concept of primary, secondary, and tertiary aging factors that can interact and heighten the risk of ADRs for the elderly patient. Primary aging factors are defined as normal physiologic changes that occur as a result of the aging process. Secondary aging factors are the changes in pathophysiology seen in the elderly which, when coupled with primary aging factors, could alter a patient's response to medication. For instance, existing disorders such as hypoxia can combine with aging changes and central nervous system drugs leading to possible altered mental status. Tertiary aging factors involve psychosocial stress (loss of income, disability, and so forth) and pharmacologic factors (possible interacting drugs). The interplay of factors could lead to a serious event. Identifying those factors that can predispose a patient to adverse drug reactions is an important way for prescribers to minimize or prevent an unwanted drug experience.

Lack of Appreciation of the Effects of Aging

The elderly frequently require reduced doses of medications, yet many health care providers do not appreciate the effects of aging on drug disposition and response. In some instances, toxicities can be attributed to accumulation of the drug in the body, secondary to failure to adjust the dosage. In order to explain and understand dosing requirements for the elderly, it is necessary to review the concepts of pharmacokinetics as they relate to the aging body.

Pharmacokinetics is the study of absorption, distribution throughout the body, and elimination of medications via the processes of metabolism and excretion. Any aging changes that affect the progress of a drug through the body can alter the amount of drug available to exert its effect. Each pharmacokinetic process is briefly presented.

Drug absorption is thought to be the least affected by the aging process. It must be stated that this is perhaps the area least studied in the literature. Several aging changes in the absorption process have been noticed. The clinical significance of these changes depends largely on the drug in question. Intestinal blood flow and motility, and gastric acid production are all decreased in the elderly. These changes could result in a delay or decrease in drug absorption.

A number of aging changes occur in body composition and size that can affect the distribution of a medication once it is absorbed. In general, elderly individuals are of smaller physical stature than the younger population. This change must be taken into account before the usual adult doses are prescribed. In addition, significant changes in body composition may lead to altered responses to a drug. Increased body fat content and decreased body water content and lean body weight occur with aging. Depending on the chemical nature of a particular medication, distribution can be affected. For example, alcohol is distributed to body water. The lessened body water content of the elderly predisposes them to enhanced ethanol (alcohol) toxicity. The elderly also can experience a decrease in the amount of albumin in the blood. Albumin is an important component of blood, often acting as a significant carrier of protein for certain drugs. If albumin is decreased, the amount of drug reaching the site of action could increase, exposing the elderly patient to increased drug effects and possible toxicity.

After the drug is distributed it is removed from the body primarily by two routes: metabolism and excretion. Hepatic (liver) metabolism as a function of age is difficult to interpret because so many other factors can influence the liver's ability to process drugs. Also, some publications present conflicting results of medications studied. Further studies will be required to determine whether human drug metabolism declines with aging.

The aging changes of renal (kidney) physiology probably are the best defined. Because so many drugs are renally excreted and there exist tools to help predict renal function, clinicians can have a great impact in this area. Rowe, Andres, Tobin, Norris, and Shock (1976) demonstrated the relationship of age to renal function in a study using males. It was shown that serum creatinine alone poorly predicts the ability to clear substances from the body. Creatinine clearance, a more accurate measure of renal function, was shown to decline with increasing age. The major disadvantage in measuring creatinine clearance is the requirement of the carefully timed urine collections. Several equations and nomograms have been used to predict creatinine clearance. One such useful equation uses a single, steady serum creatinine measurement and is based on the fact that creatinine excretion is proportional to lean body mass (which declines with age) and inversely proportional to age. Use of this method of predicting renal function can reduce significantly the possibility of drug toxicity.

In short, relatively little information is available to explain the effects of aging on drug disposition at this point in time. The need for further research in this area is obvious. Until better information is available, the need for carefully individualized therapy based on adequate knowledge of the pharmacology of drugs cannot be overemphasized.

Provider Factors that Contribute to Medication Problems in the Elderly

Much emphasis has been placed on provider-related aspects of medication problems in the elderly, particularly the lack of appreciation of age-related changes in drug elimination. It again must be emphasized that there are many reasons for medication problems or misuse, and they are not all related to the health care providers. Nevertheless, it is important to highlight key aspects of caring for the medication needs of the elderly. These aspects could serve as criteria for geriatric prescribing (Vestal, 1984). According to Vestal's suggestions for better patient-provider prescription practices, there are eight guidelines that need to be considered:

(1) Strive for a diagnosis prior to treatment;
(2) Take a careful drug history;
(3) Know the pharmacology of the drugs prescribed;
(4) Titrate the dose with patient response;
(5) Use smaller doses in the elderly;
(6) Simplify the therapeutic regimen;
(7) Regularly review the drugs in the treatment plan and discontinue those not needed; and
(8) Remember that drugs may cause illness.

Key factors from this list of guidelines are discussed next.

Proper diagnosis. An elderly person's symptoms could be the result of an adverse drug reaction or medication misuse, poor nutrition, social deprivation, or any number of reasons. An inaccurate diagnosis could possibly lead to unnecessary and even harmful drug therapy.

Drug history. A careful drug history that includes nonprescription medication information is necessary to assess the possibility of drug interactions and drug-induced symptoms of disease. Many practitioners encourage periodic "brown bag" visits to the office. During such sessions, the patient brings any and all medications to the office (often in a paper sack) for review by the physician. This can be an important tool in obtaining an accurate drug history.

Titrate the dose and simplify the regimen. Each elder's response to medications should be carefully monitored. Dosages should then be adjusted according to the patient's response. Continual review of the patient's drug regimen also provides good opportunity to eliminate unneeded drugs.

Simplify the drug regimen. Be sensitive to the special needs of an elder with impaired mental, visual, or physical function. It may be necessary to involve a friend or family member in the patient's treatment when memory is impaired. The arthritic patient may require nonchildproof containers. The stroke patient may require liquid medications if swallowing is difficult. The patient with impaired vision could benefit from adequate verbal information, reinforced with written information in large print.

SUMMARY

As the number of geriatric patients increases, the need for skilled management of this population's medication problems becomes more evident. The aged represent the largest group of prescription medication users, yet we know the least about effective use of medication among this cohort. There are many examples of medication use problems among the elderly. Some originate with patients, others with providers. Four major factors contributing to these problems are patient medication misuse, adverse drug reactions, lack of appreciation of the effects of aging, and inaccurate medical diagnosis. Most professionals believe that greater knowledge of age-related changes in physiology that may influence drug response can foster judicious use of medications in these special individuals. Thus it is incumbent upon practitioners in medicine, pharmacy, and nursing to acquire information and constantly update this as geriatric pharmaceutical research progresses.

REFERENCES

Kasper, J. A. (1982, April). *Prescribed medicines: Use, expenditures, and source of payment.* Data Preview 9, National Health Care Expenditure Study (DHHS Publication No. PHS 82-3320). Washington, DC: Government Printing Office.

Michocki, R. J., & Lamy, P. P. (1988). A risk approach to adverse drug reactions. *Journal of the American Geriatric Society, 36,* 79.

Rowe, J. W., Andres, R., Tobin, J. D., Norris, A. H., & Shock, N. W. (1976). The effect of age on creatinine clearance in men: A cross-sectional and longitudinal study. *Journal of Gerontology, 31*(2), 155.

Vestal, R. E. (1984). Geriatric clinical pharmacology: An overview. In R. E. Vestal (Ed.), *Drug treatment in the elderly.* Sydney, Australia: ADIS Health Science Press.

Chapter 4

THE EMERGENCE OF ALZHEIMER'S DISEASE
Issues and Concerns

ROSAMOND ROBBERT

Mental or cognitive problems have probably coexisted with the human race throughout history. The general history of psychiatry can be traced to Hippocrates, but the genealogy of the psychiatry of old age remains obscure and ill defined. The paucity of references to dementia or any mental conditions of the elderly in comprehensive histories of medical psychology testify to this issue. (Alexander, 1972).

Nineteenth-century physicians tended to equate dementia with the aging process. Writing in 1805, Pinel suggested that dementia was associated with aging and was therefore incurable:

> May dementia, from an occasional cause, be properly identified with that originating in old age: and are they not equally incurable? All the facts that I am acquainted with appear to countenance this melancholy truth. (Pinel, 1806, pp. 200-201)

The British practitioner Sir Henry Maudsley was less convinced that aging alone was the primary cause of dementia:

> The natural decline of the mental faculties which in greater or less degree commonly accompanies the bodily decline of old age should be distinguished from the greater loss of mental power known as senile dementia. (Maudsley, 1876, p. 254)

This question of the relationship between advancing age and dementia remains with us today. As Achenbaum notes, two schools of thought have vied for acceptance during the 20th century: "One school considered 'senility' a pathological disorder; the other described it as a normal physiological state" (Achenbaum, 1978, p. 120). Indeed, Achenbaum suggests that the course of future research in this century is less clear because we recognize the baffling complexities of senescence more sharply.

In 1906, Alois Alzheimer presented his clinical and neuropathological findings on a 51-year-old woman who had exhibited symptoms of memory loss and disorientation that were, despite his best efforts, untreatable. Alzheimer reported that autopsy data revealed pathological changes in her brain leading him to conclude that she had died of a very specific disease process. Ultimately the condition became known as Alzheimer's disease and was classified as a presenile dementia.

This classification was perhaps due to the age of Alzheimer's patient. Whatever the reason, Alzheimer's disease was regarded as a relatively rare disease entity affecting persons not yet considered to be old. Older persons suffering from cognitive loss generally were considered to be suffering from senile dementia. The first two editions of the *Diagnostic and Statistical Manual* of the American Psychiatric Association, published in 1952 and 1968, respectively, reflect this position. In addition, the disease was categorized in both manuals as a chronic or irreversible "organic brain syndrome." The third edition, published in 1980, recommended a single category to describe Alzheimer's disease to be known as Primary Degenerative Dementia of the Alzheimer Type.

The use of the term "senility" adds even more problems. Writing in 1975, Robert Butler chastised the medical profession and laity alike for the use of "senility" as both a diagnosis and a lay term for any older person displaying minimal symptoms of forgetfulness. The use of the term justifies therapeutic nihilism because therapists then "need not undertake the kind of careful diagnostic assessment needed to determine a proper course of treatment" (Butler, 1975, p. 232).

In apparent frustration at the confusion in terminology, Lissy Jarvik proposed yet another term:

> I propose the term *paraskepsia* to describe the cognitive impairment independent of etiology. Derived from the Greek words *para,* meaning "alongside," and *skepsia,* meaning "thought," paraskepsia means thought which is at the end of, or alongside, ordinary thought. Paraskepsia does not imply etiology and, even more significantly, it does not imply that the thought processes are inadequate for all life situations. Calling someone a paraskeptic would not have the pejorative connotation of calling that person demented. (Jarvik, 1982, p. 106)

Perhaps, fortunately, her suggestion appears not to have been accorded much attention. Currently, the preferred terminology for cognitive loss in older persons appears to be Senile Dementia of the Alzheimer's Type (SDAT) or, more basically, Alzheimer's disease.

Today Alzheimer's disease is no longer considered to be a rare disease but rather is said to be perhaps the fourth leading cause of death among elderly persons. Writing in 1984, Butler described some of the strategies involved in achieving this change in definition.

THE DISCOVERY OF ALZHEIMER'S DISEASE

Dr. Robert Butler was appointed the first director of the newly established National Institute on Aging in 1976. The mandate of the institute was to promote research on aging. His first major responsibility was to develop a research agenda, to which he responded by making a critical decision to target Alzheimer's disease as a major initiative for the National Institute on Aging.

One of the first initiatives was to sponsor an international workshop conference in 1978 for researchers and practitioners interested in the cognitive problems of old age. This conference was, in Butler's opinion, of "catalytic importance" in many ways (Butler, 1984, p. 33). The attendees generally agreed that the categorization of Alzheimer's disease should include both senile and presenile dementias, a reformulation that expanded the epidemiological base from a few rare cases to one of potentially millions.

Ultimately the problem became, however, one of promotion:

> The question was, how to make it attractive for members of the appropriations committees in Congress. How do you sell Alzheimer's Disease? One public relations expert told me we should change the name. I considered this poor

advice. I turned to the director of the information office, Jan Shure, . . . and working together we developed successive steps to raise public consciousness about "senility" and Alzheimer's Disease. It was my judgment that Congress would respond to an increasing popular awareness of the problem, to public testimony and to behind-the-scenes discussions. (Butler, 1984, pp. 33-34)

Together with his director of information, Butler developed strategies to communicate with not only the medical community and Congress, but also the general public. Congressional hearings were developed, publications were stimulated in professional journals, the media were utilized. In addition, families of Alzheimer's victims were contacted:

I learned that support groups for families with an Alzheimer's victim existed in various cities. In 1979 we invited them to Bethesda. Concerned that there not be a splintering of groups competing over precious dollars and incipient public support, we urged the establishment of a national federation. (Butler, 1984, p. 34)

One year later, in 1980, the Alzheimer's Disease and Related Disorders Association was established.

Butler concludes that the Alzheimer's story can be seen as politics at its best:

Health-science policy was [being] directed toward something very important. Often scientists are negative toward politics, towards advocacy and toward communicating with the public. However, it is the public that suffers and the public that pays the bill for science and for medical and related services. It seems more than appropriate that physicians and medical scientists in general play a major role in advancing the public's understanding of a specific disease. (Butler, 1984, p. 34)

As a result of this remarkable initiative and collaboration, Alzheimer's has become a household word. Indeed, the "Alzheimer's movement" provides us with a model for expanding public policy in a variety of ways, not the least of which is in long-term care. Given the increased awareness of today, it is essential that professionals working with older persons and their families be familiar with the multiple issues connected with the social, psychosocial, behavioral, and medical aspects of Alzheimer's disease as it impacts the victims, their families, and social institutions—most particularly the service delivery system.

Underlying all concerns, however, whether they are related to basic science, social policy, or family dynamics, is the critical need for an appropriate diagnostic assessment. Recognition of the importance of diagnosis basically has emerged together with the perception of Alzheimer's disease as a social and medical problem. It appears, however, that knowledge of the importance of diagnosis and appropriate evaluative processes is not yet as widely understood as it should be.

During the course of presenting many workshops and courses on Alzheimer's disease, I have been amazed by the number of people who assume that their family member is suffering from Alzheimer's disease when no evaluation has been made. They have, in effect, exchanged "senility" for "Alzheimer's disease" with no behavioral change on their part other than the use of the new label. Conversely, I still hear stories about short consultations with physicians ending in a diagnosis of Alzheimer's disease. Equally disturbing are the numbers of professionals observed attending educational forums who have little or no knowledge of the recommended diagnostic workup for someone suspected of having Alzheimer's disease. These have included social workers, nurses, and many paraprofessionals.

DIAGNOSIS OF ALZHEIMER'S DISEASE

Proper identification of the disease is crucial to management. Indeed, there is an ethical responsibility for those involved since there are potentially reversible conditions whose symptoms mimic a true dementia.

At the present time a diagnosis of Alzheimer's disease can only be confirmed at autopsy. The diagnostic effort, therefore, is characterized as a "rule out" process. The diagnosis of Alzheimer's disease was described by Wells in 1979 as diagnosis by default: "Demented patients in whom no specific cause . . . can be found should, then, generally be considered to have Alzheimer's disease" (Wells, 1979, p. 519). Despite efforts to develop a definitive diagnostic instrument or protocol, Wells's admonition remains valid today.

Error rates in diagnosis are largely unknown; however, several behavioral factors have been suggested that contribute to diagnostic error. These include: ageism (neglect caused by expectations that the patient is merely "senile"); failure to use strict diagnostic criteria; insufficient time devoted to obtaining a history or examining patients; absence of a policy of searching for reversible causes of the confusion; inadequate recourse to special tests; incompatibility between the diagnostician and the patient due to cultural or educational background (Gurland & Toner, 1985).

The initial evaluation for suspected Alzheimer's disease is relatively straightforward. The following discussion is taken from a *Conference State-*

ment on the Differential Diagnosis of Dementing Diseases published by the National Institutes of Health in 1987. The authors of this document stress that the diagnostic workup is time consuming, but nothing else can replace it.

The *history* is a most important component of the initial evaluation. This should be obtained from family members most responsible for and in contact with the patient. In addition, the patient himself or herself should be involved in this process whenever possible. A chronological account of the patient's current problems should include a description of the mode of onset and an in-depth description of behavioral issues. Previous medical records should also be consulted. The medical history should include questions about relevant systemic disease, trauma, surgery, psychiatric disorders, nutrition, alcohol and/or substance abuse, exposure to environmental toxins, and the use of prescription and nonprescription medications. The significance of behavioral changes should be evaluated within the context of the patient's social, ethnic, racial, educational, occupational, marital, and family background.

Screening for mental status is essential. Users of mental status tests such as the Mini-Mental-State are warned, however, that they carry a relatively high risk of both false positives and missed cases. Short screening batteries that require a longer time are more satisfactory. Examples of such short batteries are the Washington University SDAT Screening Battery and the Iowa Screening Battery for Mental Decline. These tests are used not only to establish baseline data but also to evaluate change over time. They should, therefore, be administered on a regular basis. The reader is warned, however, that a patient should not be considered demented solely on the basis of a poor score on a mental status test. Changes that normally occur must be understood and taken into consideration. Age-associated memory impairment is a controversial condition that may be merely a manifestation of normal age-related changes in memory.

Diagnostic tests are recommended as follows with modifications made on the basis of individual circumstances:

(1) Complete blood count
(2) Electrolyte panel
(3) Screening metabolic panel
(4) Thyroid function tests
(5) Vitamin B_{12} and folate levels
(6) Tests for syphilis and, depending on history, for human immunodeficiency antibodies
(7) Urinanalysis

(8)   Electrocardiogram

(9)   Chest X-ray

In addition the following recommendations are made:

> Computed tomography of the brain (without contrast) is appropriate in the presence of history suggestive of a mass, or focal neurological signs, or in dementia of brief duration. Unless such diagnosis is obvious on first contact, computed tomography should be done. Magnetic resonance imaging is more sensitive than computed tomography for detection of small infarcts, mass lesions, atrophy of the brain stem, and other subcortical structures; it may also clarify ambiguous computed tomography findings. Inexperienced interpreters may make too much of ambiguous or nonspecific findings on magnetic resonance imaging.

As noted above, the diagnostic process requires investigating other illnesses and conditions that may be causal factors. Numerous studies warn against confusing a true dementia with a potentially reversible condition. These conditions are often referred to as "pseudodementias."

Arrestable or reversible causes of dementia include *intoxications*. Medications capable of producing dementia include the increasing large number of neuroactive and psychoactive agents, the opiate analgesics, and the adrenocortical steroids.

Any *infection* capable of involving the brain is capable of producing dementing illness. Many cases of dementia are prevented from happening in the first place by the effective treatment of leptomeningitis and encephalitis.

Metabolic disorders of, for example, the thyroid, parathyroid, adrenals, and pituitary generally are reversible. Without identification these conditions may exhibit symptoms of dementia.

Nutritional disorders related to alcoholism potentially can be controlled. Korsakoff's dementia, related to alcoholism, once established, may undergo a degree of remission, but the pathological changes are irreversible.

Vascular disorders, such as severe hypertension, are one of the most frequent causes of dementia. Cardiac disease also produces dementia by single or repeated episodes of cerebral ischemia and hypoxia due to acute or intermittent disorders of cardiac function.

(The reader is reminded that the above discussion stems largely from the *Consensus Statement* developed as a result of a conference convened by the National Institutes of Health in July 1987.)

DEPRESSION AS A PSEUDODEMENTIA

Roth (1981) points to the critical issue of differentiating depression from dementia. He emphasizes the problems in so doing and notes that it is important to observe the patient over time and not to rush to a hasty diagnosis. More particularly, he suggests that the ability to perform complex skills tends to be retained in depression and is not generally observed in dementia. (See also Caine, 1981; Kral, 1983; Reifler, Larson, & Hanley, 1982.) Gurland and Toner (1983) found that the depressed older person can be confused. Depressive episodes may be associated with sleep disorders, a loss of appetite, and weight loss, all of which can contribute to confused behavior. In addition, the authors note that there was a tendency in their subjects to only report physical symptoms and to mask or fail to report psychic pain.

Writing in 1986, Blazer suggests that, paradoxically, depression in older persons gives the practitioner a cause for hope. He points to depression as a treatable illness. Even when compounded with the early stages of a true dementia, if recognized, it can be treated. The differential diagnosis involves using screening tests for depression; history taking, including life- style and family dynamics; and basic laboratory tests. Sleep studies where possible can augment the diagnostic process. As Blazer notes, however:

> The medical, psychological and psychiatric workup of the depressed older adult is complex, increasingly sophisticated, but nevertheless not 100 percent accurate. More often than clinicians wish to admit, time is the true indicator of the nature, extent and characteristics of depressive symptomatology. (Blazer, 1986, p. 23)

Despite the complexities of differentiating depression from dementia, Blazer concludes that no health problem in later life deserves therapeutic optimism more than depression since the depressive disorders of old age are treatable. Frequently they are chronic only because therapeutic intervention is not prescribed or available.

In 1976, Katzman emphasized the importance of diagnosis in suspected cases of dementia: "It is a truly terrible diagnostic error to overlook the possibility of a reversible dementia, yet it is variously estimated that between twenty and thirty percent of patients with chronic brain syndrome are misdiagnosed" (Katzman, 1976, p. 217).

As noted, the error rate in diagnosis is not known. The diagnosis of dementia, however, has become more sophisticated and hopefully more accurate in the intervening years since Katzman raised his concern. Knowledge of potentially reversible conditions also is improving. Because serious implications are inherent in the diagnostic process, it is the responsibility not only of those directly involved in the process, but also of all professionals and lay persons serving elderly confused persons, to be informed of the current state of knowledge so that we may advocate on their behalf. Every person suspected of having Alzheimer's disease deserves the most sophisticated assessment currently available.

REFERENCES

Achenbaum, W. A. (1978). *Old age in the new land: The American experience since 1790.* Baltimore, MD: Johns Hopkins University Press.

Alexander, D. A. (1972). Senile dementia: A changing perspective. *British Journal of Psychiatry, 121,* 207-214.

American Psychiatric Association. (1952). *Diagnostic and statistical manual of mental disorders* (1st ed.). Washington, DC: Author.

American Psychiatric Association. (1968). *Diagnostic and statistical manual of mental disorders* (2nd ed.). Washington, DC: Author.

Blazer, D. (1986). Depression: Paradoxically, a cause for hope. *Generations, 10,*(3), 21-23.

Butler, R. N. (1975). *Why survive? Being old in America.* New York: Harper & Row.

Butler, R. N. (1984). How Alzheimer's became a public issue. *Generations, 9*(1), 33-35.

Caine, E. D. (1981). Pseudodementia: Current concepts and future directions. *Archives of General Psychiatry, 38* 1359-1364.

Gurland, B., & Toner, J. (1985). Differentiating dementia from non-dementing conditions. In R. Mayeux & W. G. Rosen (Eds.), *Advances in neurology.* New York: Raven.

Jarvik, L. (1982). Dementia in old age: Reflections on nomenclature. *Psychiatric Clinics of North America, 5*(1), 105-106.

Katzman, R. (1976). The prevalence and malignancy of Alzheimer's disease. *Archives of Neurology, 33,* 217-218.

Kral, V. A. (1983). The relationship between senile dementia (Alzheimer type) and depression. *Canadian Journal of Psychiatry, 28,* 304-306.

Maudsley, H. (1876). Responsibility in mental diseases. In D. N. Robinson (Ed.), *Significant contributions to the history of psychology* (pp. 1750-1920). Washington, DC: University Publications of America.

National Institutes of Health. (1987). *Differential diagnosis of dementing diseases: Conference statement, 6*(11), 1-8.

Pinel, P. (1806). A treatise on insanity. In D. N. Robinson (Ed.), *Significant contributions to the history of psychology* (pp. 1750-1920). Washington, DC: University Publications of America.

Reifler, B. V., Larson, E., & Hanley, R. (1982). Coexistence of cognitive impairment and depression in geriatric outpatients. *American Journal of Psychiatry, 139,* 623-626.

Roth, M. (1981). The diagnosis of dementia in late and middle life. In J. A. Mortimer & L. M. Schuman (Eds.), *The epidemiology of dementia.* Oxford: Oxford University Press.

Wells, C. E. (1979). Diagnosis of dementia. *Psychomatics, 20*(8), 517-522.

Chapter 5

THE OLDER ADULT ALCOHOLIC CLIENT

NOVA MUIR GREEN
JANET D. BRIDGHAM

Alcoholism among older adults is a leading concern to health care providers. It is conservatively estimated that three million adults 65 years of age or older have alcohol-related problems. Some nursing homes report that as many as half of their patients have lost the ability to live independently because of alcohol abuse resulting in severe memory impairment, confusion, and loss of mobility caused by falls. As the number of aging adults dramatically increases so should interest in assessing the relationship between aging and alcohol abuse, and finding effective methods of treatment and prevention. Through our work with older adults in a hospital setting, we have encountered many persons with dependency problems with alcohol or prescription drugs. We have come to believe that the use of alcohol presents special hazards to persons in the last third of the life span. In this chapter, we will present information about older alcoholics and include our professional experiences and opinions.

PREVALENCE OF ALCOHOL ABUSE

Statistics regarding elderly alcoholics vary from one study to another, and assertions that seem valid in relation to one observed group are disclaimed or modified by observations of another (Blose, 1978; Bozzetti & MacMurray, 1977; Maletta, 1982). One point of agreement in most studies is that alcoholism among older adults is underreported. Problems with alcohol are said to account for 12% of male and 4% of female admissions of patients over age 60 to inpatient psychiatric facilities, and an even larger percentage of admissions to outpatient mental health programs (Bozzetti & MacMurray, 1977; Maletta, 1982; Pascarelli, 1974; Zimberg, 1987). Hospital admission studies of older adults have found that 20% to 60% of these patients have alcohol problems in addition to the problems for which they are being hospitalized, with the cause-and-effect relationship undetermined (Maletta, 1982). It has been believed that alcohol abuse peaks between the ages of 35 and 50 and then declines with increasing age (Cahalan, Cisin, & Crossley, 1974). Recently, this has been questioned as some studies show incidence rates peaking twice, at ages 45 to 55 (23 cases per 1,000) and again at ages 65 to 74 (21 cases per 1,000); elderly widows show the extraordinary rate of 105 cases per 1,000 (Bozzetti & MacMurray, 1977; Maletta, 1982).

DENIAL OF THE PROBLEM

Collection of valid statistics is impaired because of belated recognition of alcohol addiction among older adults. Much of this is due to denial of the problem. Zimberg (1987) states

> The delayed perception of this subpopulation of alcoholics includes the more subtle manifestations of alcoholism in the elderly and a greater denial of its existence by health care professionals and family members because of philosophical bias. Most health professionals and family members of the elderly alcoholics dismiss the problem by rationalizing that elderly persons have nothing left except their bottle, so why take that away. This view reflects rejection of the elderly by our youth-oriented culture. (p. 58)

Maletta (1982) points to the professional's reluctance to ask questions of the elderly person and to relative lack of visibility after retirement. In contrast with younger alcoholics who come to the attention of traffic police and courts, employers, and family problem counselors, older alcoholics "primarily come to the attention of medical hospitals, where a disease of the specific organ system rather than the whole person is usually treated" (Maletta, 1982, p. 779).

The older individual also may deny the problem. None of our clients have been self-referred. Rather, they are found and referred by in-home health care workers, visiting nurses, hospital social workers and discharge planners, adult children, inpatient substance abuse centers for follow-up, and probation officers who do not like to send elderly alcoholics to jail. These casefinders provide the impetus needed to get the older adult alcoholic into treatment, as these clients typically have little self-motivation toward treatment because of denial, or from ignorance and feelings of hopelessness about their condition. Often, our clients seem to consent to treatment as an act of courtesy and/or gratitude to us or to the casefinder for the affection and concern shown to them. It has been stated by other workers, and we agree, that "Motivation to stop drinking does not cause a person to go into treatment. It is a process which happens in treatment" (Flynn-Breeden, 1988).

CRITERIA FOR THE LABEL "ALCOHOLIC"

People typically resist being called "alcoholic." The definition many persons, including our clients, often use considers the amount of liquor that should be consumed. There is great debate about this and the severity of social and physical problems required in order to fit that category. The American Medical Association in 1956, in contrast to the then-prevailing attitude that alcoholism indicated a flawed moral character (Plunkett & Brock, 1956, p. 750), defined alcoholism as a disease. The AMA definition emphasizes the symptom of immediate or progressive loss of control over drinking behavior. Similarly, the *Diagnostic and Statistical Manual of Mental Disorders*, Third Edition (DSM-III), defines substance *dependence* as loss of control of drinking behavior shown by unsuccessful attempts to regain control, and obsessive use despite legal, moral, social or occupational offenses and sanctions, and adds the criteria of high physical tolerance or (late) sudden loss of tolerance for the substance. DSM-III distinguishes between dependence and substance *abuse*. The criteria for substance abuse include "continued use despite. . . persistent or recurrent social, occupational, psychological or physical problem(s) . . . caused or exacerbated by use" or use in physically hazardous situations, for example, driving while drunk (American Psychiatric Association, 1980, p. 109). In a Leader's Guide for group education and discussion about alcohol, the National Council on Alcohol (NCA) clarifies the definition of the loss of control:

> The alcoholic may be able to have one or two drinks on occasion, and then stop. But s/he can never guarantee how much s/he will drink, once s/he begins to drink. . . . a person who stops drinking for a period of time, who moves to get away from drinking friends, changes jobs or friends or type of alcohol (from gin, vodka to beer or wine) is trying to regain control. "Social Drinkers" do not have to do this.

Once acquired, the disease of alcoholism is usually defined as incurable but can be arrested through abstinence from alcohol.

CAUSES OF ALCOHOL ABUSE

Some researchers have suggested that alcohol abuse by older adults may have several causes. For some it does not indicate loss of control of drinking but a self-medicating response to the losses and stresses of aging. It is assumed that these persons, "late onset" alcohol abusers, will decrease their drinking when some of the stresses of aging are alleviated (Zimberg, 1987). Maletta (1982) cautions that "the concomitance of life problems and substance abuse in the same elderly individual is no proof that one caused the other" (p. 784). He further warns that, "From a psychotherapeutic viewpoint, it might be suggested that the belief that there is no other way for depressed old people to cope other than by means of alcohol may in fact be a *counter-transference problem based on the observer's perception of old age*" (Maletta, 1982, p. 784) (emphasis in original).

We reviewed our clients on the "early onset/late onset" dimension and found about the same proportion as some other studies: one third of our clients reported that their drinking became a problem after retirement, and two thirds started drinking heavily in their middle forties or earlier. None of our clients, however, were nondrinkers before retirement, and about one third of those who started drinking heavily in their thirties and forties described it as a self-medicating response—personal problems triggered the increase in their drinking. Almost without exception, our clients said they also used alcohol for "fun," to increase their pleasure and relaxation. This age group used alcohol for the same reason as other age groups, as a socially appropriate and acceptable method to medicate sadness and to increase sociability, enjoyment, and happiness. Over time, varying in length for different individuals, they lost the ability to choose when and how much they drank.

Indeed, an ongoing problem for our clients (which never goes away) is how to stay away from those glamorized, seductive, ubiquitous symbols of the good life—wine, whiskey, and beer! Relapse usually is estimated at 40%, and our experience supports that figure. Our frustration with relapse makes us wish (a) that the sale of alcohol could be restricted to liquor stores, to help our recovering clients resist impulse buying when they are first learning how to stay sober, and (b) that alcohol would develop the taint of social disapproval now associated with tobacco. We have clients who argue "if alcohol was really bad for your health, it would say so on the bottle." We have also heard client comments such as "I never drank as much as they do on the soap operas. . . . I don't see how those people stay on their feet!"

It is worth noticing that these clients were *not* socialized to believe that cocaine and marijuana are acceptable ways to medicated sorrow and increase happiness, and they do not use these drugs. Most, in fact, tend to be highly critical of people who do use them, and only admit on reflection, ". . . although I guess I'm just as bad." Our particular group of clients thought they were acting "just like everybody else." They did not fear the effects of alcohol nor anticipate the possibility of addiction. Over and over, they express wonder and surprise, "How did it happen?"

Boredom is another possibility. As George Bernard Shaw wrote, "A perpetual holiday is a good working definition of hell." Shaw was probably a workaholic, but he was surely not the first nor last person to find free time a burden. A study on alcohol use and social interaction in retirement communities by Alexander and Duff (1988) supports the hypothesis that alcoholism among older adults can develop independent of aging problems of poverty, bereavement, and isolation. The study subjects were white, prosperous, middle-class men and women in three retirement communities, with a median income of $20,055 and a median age of 75.6, with an age range of 57 to 97 years. The findings suggest that

> The quantity of drinking [was] found to be positively associated with higher levels of social interaction. . . . Socially isolated individuals were more likely to be non-drinkers and less likely to be heavy drinkers than gregarious residents. . . . The majority of heavy drinkers in the community admitted that they drank alone as well as with others. *Furthermore, the most socially active individuals were also the most likely to drink alone. It seems that even for the highly social heavy drinkers, their drinking is more than a social activity.* (pp. 634-635) (emphasis in original.)

The authors further found that

> The social life of the community encouraged residents to drink as part of the process of integration into the leisure subculture. Twenty-three percent of the total sample and 29 percent of the most socially active said that they felt there were some groups in the community in which people had to drink to feel accepted. (p. 635)

Our clients' most stressful physical, social, and psychological problems clearly are related to their alcoholism. They also have age-related problems; but rather than abusing alcohol because they cannot cope with these problems, the cause-and-effect relationship seems to be reversed, best described by an Alcoholics Anonymous motto, "There is no problem so bad that alcohol can't make it worse!" We have been thrilled and astonished by the extraordinary improvement in physical health, mood, and ability to cope with problems that occurs when clients are completely detoxified. The "alcoholic personality," dependent, self-pitying, manipulative, and mendacious, seems to be created by the drug alcohol. When our clients are detoxified, they no longer share a "personality." Individual tastes, values, attitudes, and abilities emerge, especially the ability to cope with many of the problems of aging that were overwhelming before sobriety.

We are not asserting here that our clients have no problems other than alcohol addiction. Like nonalcoholic older adults, they have experienced physical, social, and financial losses, and have at least as much difficulty finding a life-style in retirement that fits their abilities and satisfies their need to be useful and happy. We also agree with those who attribute alcoholism to the stresses of aging that the probability of maintaining sobriety is greatly enhanced when our clients find a satisfying life-style in which to invest time and energy. Our observations of our clients lead us to believe, however, that they became addicted to alcohol *not* because of the unique problems of aging but because of their reaction to the unique properties of alcohol. Physical changes from aging intensify the effect of alcohol, and the aging body is not as efficient at detoxification. The older person has time to fill, usually without constraining social responsibilities, and alcohol never fails to relieve boredom and kill time.

Alcohol is used, by people of all ages, to induce feelings of pleasure in leisure situations that sober judgment might assess as boring or tedious. The lack of interesting activities and responsibilities after retirement, and the long hours to fill, may be important factors in the increase of drinking among older adults, with an associated increase in the development of alcohol dependence.

SPECIAL PROBLEMS WITH DIAGNOSIS

It has been estimated that of the older alcoholics who became ill enough to be placed in nursing homes, 60% are diagnosed with organic brain syndrome. This may be a misdiagnosis due to the length of time necessary for an older adult to completely detoxify from the effect of alcohol. The older adult may still be confused and unsteady after the standard detoxification treatment has been completed. The signs and symptoms typical of alcoholism--depression, incompetence, incontinence, and confusion—are stereotypical symptoms of aging. In a younger person, these symptoms would stimulate immediate concern and action. In an older person, they may be dismissed as signs of senility. Misdiagnosis of the potentially reversible condition of alcoholism may sentence the elderly alcoholic to a half-life in an institution where he or she remains incompetent on sedative drugs that have the same effect as alcohol.

A cultural myth that interferes with accurate diagnosis is the belief that aging itself is a tragic disease, to which depression is a logical response. As one comedian expressed it, "If you're not miserable, you're not paying attention!" One of our clients had been drinking, weeping, and sweating copiously for 14 years. Her doctor suspected, but had not addressed, the excessive drinking problem. Her labile emotional state was attributed to an inability to adjust to retirement, and the sweating was blamed on "pain from arthritic knees." In a younger woman, it might have been noted much earlier that the patient's medical history showed the onset of these symptoms coinciding with a hysterectomy operation. When this client received estrogen therapy, she was able to stay serene and dry, inside and out.

Another client was misdiagnosed with organic brain syndrome because he was still confused and unable to maintain walking equilibrium after the traditional number of days in detoxification. Through the efforts of his therapist and his family, he was transferred to another treatment center where detoxification procedures were continued. He made a total recovery. This case was a powerful example to everyone concerned that older adults may require several weeks or even months to recover from the physical effects of alcohol. The aging body clears the toxins more slowly, but it can recover with enough time and the right regimen.

SPECIAL PROBLEMS WITH TREATMENT

One of the common myths of aging, "You can't teach an old dog new tricks," has been applied to the older alcoholic. We were told recently by a substance abuse counselor, "After age 60, alcoholics don't recover." It is frustrating to treat addicts of any age because of the high incidence of relapse, but there is no evidence at all that older adults are uniquely impervious to recovery. Maletta (1982) observes that

> There seems to be a prevailing attitude held by many that with elderly individuals it is useless to attempt to actively treat biopsychosocial problems, including those of alcohol abuse. It is as though when an individual reaches a certain point in life, the cost of being treated becomes greater than the benefit to be accrued. (p. 789)

Reluctance to treat older adult alcoholics seems to reflect not only a negative attitude about the social value of the client but also feelings of revulsion and distaste toward that life stage. Zimberg (1987) refers to this attitude of distaste as the "philosophical bias" that generates the comment that "elderly persons have nothing left but their bottles, so why take that away." This view of the last third of the life cycle, the years from 60 to 90, can discourage both therapist and client. Carl Eisdorfer comments that "The expectancy that aging brings inevitable decline, depression, and disability has led to an unwarranted therapeutic nihilism" (Eisdorfer, Cohen & Veith, 1980, p. 7). In a senior workshop discussion, one participant expressed his dislike of all the terms used to describe his age group—Senior Citizens, Golden Oldies, Older Adults, and so forth. He said, "They keep changing the name but they never come up with a good one!" The group came to the conclusion that the name would never be appealing until the people so described valued their condition. One spokesperson declared, "We are the ones who have to make our later years golden!"

Treatment really begins for the older adult alcoholic when someone values him or her enough to try to interrupt the destructive drinking. Contrary to the assumption implicit in ". . . don't take the bottle away!", addiction to alcohol is not a comfortable or happy condition. Recovering older adults have described their feelings as shame, despair, self-hatred, and hopelessness. The casefinder represents hope. When we meet our client, we try to project our belief, acquired through experience, that recovery from alcoholism is possible, and problems that seem insurmountable while drinking deflate amazingly when the person becomes sober.

Particular treatment recommendations depend on the individual client, but the majority of our clients either have been to an inpatient treatment center or we recommend that they enter one for detoxification and education about alcohol in a protected environment. Clients vary in their resistance to inpatient treatment, depending, it seems, on the comfort of their current living situation. The client who is isolated and uncared for, or who is on the verge of being evicted, has a more positive view of inpatient treatment than the client whose income or caretakers protect him or her from the more extreme unpleasant consequences of addiction.

MAKING A CASE FOR ABSTINENCE

We teach the disease concept of alcoholism and recommend abstinence as essential to recovery. Abstinence is a controversial treatment recommendation. Some therapists report a successful return to moderate alcohol use among alcoholic clients in programs that reduce some of the social and psychological stress of aging (Zimberg, 1987). Others describe, with enthusiasm and conviction worthy of a member of La Leche League, the psychological, nutritional, and medical value of alcohol for the elderly, and advocate the goal of controlled drinking. One such enthusiast (Kastenbaum, 1988) cited Luigi Cornaro, author of *The Art of Living Long,* as a model for the use of alcohol to improve aging:

> As a mature person, [Cornara] found the moderate use of wine in appropriate circumstances to be an enhancement to a balanced life in which exercise, work, and social responsibility all played significant roles. . . . Cornaro . . . personally discovered both the hazards and satisfactions of alcoholic beverages. (p. 68)

It is fairly easy to provide the wine to older adults in nursing homes, but the balance—the appropriate and satisfying "exercise, work, and social responsibility"—is not as easy to find. Perhaps the behavioral improvements noted in studies where alcohol was added to the nursing home diet may have indicated the "halo effect" of unusual attention, interest, and approval accorded to study subjects. In any case, we assert that ingestion of an addictive drug that depresses judgment is risk-taking behavior at any age, but for the older adult, even moderate amounts of alcohol can have serious negative consequences. If the older adult is depressed or has suffered the loss of a friend or spouse, alcohol will increase the depression and interface with the process of grieving. With consistent use of alcohol, an individual can remain in a state of unresolved grieving for 20 years or longer, and we have clients who have done this. Small amounts of alcohol can interfere with sleeping patterns, impair memory, reduce fine muscle coordination, and disturb equilibrium. A recent study (Gold, Ahern, & Miller, 1988) analyzing 10 million prescription claims found that 27 of the 30 prescription drugs most frequently purchased by older adults are considered to be a alcohol-interactive. The study also noted that nearly half of the subjects who took medication with alcohol-interactive properties "rated as of major or moderate clinical significance" said that neither their physician nor pharmacist warned them to avoid alcohol. Whether their complaint shows ignorance or denial, the study indicates another serious health hazard associated with alcohol and further justifies our prejudice for abstinence.

PROBLEM IDENTIFICATION AND PROBLEM SOLVING

The productive use of leisure time has often been identified as a problem for every age group. It is our observation that our clients developed serious health and social problems by overusing alcohol—a socially acceptable, addictive, depressant drug--to medicate sadness and solve the problem of leisure. Leisure time that extends two or three days a week and four to six weeks a year is experienced as a blessing, but we do not know how to enjoy 30 years of "nothing to do." In the *Psychology of Aging,* Eisdorfer, Cohen, and Veith note that there is no role for the aged in our society. They state that, "Any system that cuts persons off from social participation at an arbitrary age not only risks losing considerable talent but creates serious new problems. . . . For many aged, retirement is a job and being a patient becomes a major social role" (p. 7). They believe that the attitude of society toward the aged will determine whether this group will be a blessing or a curse.

> To a considerable extent, the aged play the role that they and society choose for them. . . . [A] view of the aged as an experienced, motivated, and potentially participating group could profoundly influence the future treatment of older persons. . . . The aged are growing in numbers and proportion of our society. Their fate depends on whether they are viewed as a major resource or as a problem. If we stimulate reinvestment in the aged, if we recognize their potential as producers of goods and services, and as consumers, and if we provide options to the aged, we will not only significantly reduce emerging problems, but we will also address some of society's immediate problems. (p. 7-8)

A permissive attitude toward the overuse of alcohol by older adults (as implied by comments such as, "Don't take the bottle away because that's all they have left," clearly expresses a view of the elderly as a problem rather than a resource. Eisdorfer predicts that if we maintain this view, we will create a self-fulfilling prophecy, with the result that, "additional expenditures will be necessary to warehouse a group of people that, in a peculiar perversion of logic, we hope to join" (Eisdorfer, Cohen, & Veith, 1980, p. 8).

The extract above states that role definitions for older adults are determined by society and the older person. We consider this our clients' task, to reassess who they are, what they want that they can have, and how they can get it. As in every other age and situation of their lives, our clients have limits and opportunities, strengths and weaknesses to assess and use. When the recognize and accept the responsibility for inventing a life to enjoy, they think of things that did not occur to us, and move in directions we did not expect. Our treatment involves individual weekly counseling sessions that give clients an opportunity to express anxieties, resolve resentments, and make plans. We explore former and/or potential interests and desires, and how to achieve them. We strongly advocate attending Alcoholics Anonymous (A.A.) meetings, especially an older adult group initiated by clients from our program, where similar problems can be discussed and the language is more restrained. Our referral suggestions for mobile clients include social groups, other A.A. groups, senior centers, volunteer programs, senior employment agencies, community college courses, and other community activities. Homebound clients are made aware that peer counselors, senior companions, and senior home companions are available to make visits to them and provide a variety of services. We inform them of Meals on Wheels and community transportation capabilities. We are presently trying to solve space and transportation problems to be able to offer therapy group experiences to our clients.

Clark and Anderson (1967) define successful aging as the accomplishment of a set of adaptive tasks: (a) recognition of the fact of aging and instrumental limitations; (b) redefinition of physical and social life space; (c) substitution of alternative sources of need satisfaction; (d) reassessment of criteria determining self-esteem; and (e) reintegration of values and life goals. We believe that these adaptive tasks have to be accomplished at every major life change, from infancy to childhood, childhood to adolescence, adolescence to young adulthood, and young adulthood to mature middle age. The reason it is not clear how to accomplish these tasks at "young old age" and "old old age" is because we have not been there before. We have a new third of life that can be viewed as not as a punishment but as a reward.

SUMMARY

Older adults who are alcoholic often have the same problems as other adults in this life stage, complicated by some chemical problem-solving that did not work out. They may, or may not, have a history of alcohol abuse.

Among our older adult alcoholic clients we hear comments like, "Look at George Burns! He says he has five martinis a day and he's working at 90!" Sorry, Charlie. Not all of us can find enough work and responsibility to balance that many martinis! Despite the complaints, it has been our experience that when our clients are physically and mentally recovered from the effects of alcohol, they have the resources and creativity to put together a good life. We believe that it is possible to adapt to the last third of life in the same way we adapt to the losses, gains, freedoms, and responsibilities that came earlier. But we would advocate for sparkling water rather than sparkling wine to accompany the feast of later life.

REFERENCES

Alexander, F., & Duff, R. W. (1988). Social interaction and alcohol use in retirement communities. *The Gerontologist, 28*(5), 632-636.

American Psychiatric Association. (1980). *Diagnostic and statistical manual of mental disorders* (3rd ed.). Washington, DC: Author.

Bailey, M. B., Haberman, P. W., & Alksne, H. (1965). The epidemiology of alcoholism in an urban residential area. *Quarterly Journal of Studies on Alcohol, 26*, 19-40.

Blose, I. L. (1978). The relationship of alcohol to aging and the elderly. *Alcoholism Clinical and Experimental Research, 2*, 17-21.

Bozzetti, L. P., & MacMurray, J. P. (1977). Drug misuse among the elderly: A hidden meance. *Psychiatric Annual, 7*, 95-107.

Cahalan, D., Cisin, I. A., & Crossley, H. M. (1974). *American drinking practices: A national survey of drinking behavior and attitudes.* New Brunswick, NJ: Rutgers University, Rutgers Center of Alcohol Studies.

Clark, M., & Anderson, B. C. (1967). *Culture and aging.* Springfield, IL: Charles C Thomas.

Eisendorfer, C., Cohen, D., & Veith, R. (1980). The psychopathology of aging. *Current concepts, a scope publication.* The Upjohn Company.

Flynn-Breeden, L. (1988, September). *Motivating older adults into treatment.* Paper presented at the conference, Network: Older adult substance abuse services. Ann Arbor, MI.

Gold, C. H., Ahern, F. M., & Miller, S. H. (1988, October). Alcohol and prescription drug interaction: Factors associated with risk, knowledge and compliance behaviors among the elderly [Special issue]. *The Gerontologist, 28*,(238A).

Kastenbaum, R. (1988, Summer). In moderation [Special issue]. *Generations/Alcohol and Drugs.*

Maletta, G. J. (1982). Alcoholism and the aged. In E. M. Pattison & E. Kaufman (Eds.), *Encyclopedic handbook of alcoholism.* New York: Gardner.

Pascarelli, E. F. (1974). Drug dependence: An age-old problem compounded by old age. *Geriatrics, 29*, 109-114.

Plunkett, R., & Brock, M. (1956, October 20). Hospitalization of patients with alcoholism. *Journal of the American Medical Association*, p. 750.

Zimberg, S. (1987). Alcohol abuse among the elderly. In L. L. Carstensen & B. A. Edelstein (Eds.), *Handbook of clinical gerontology.* New York: Pergamon.

Chapter 6

ELDER ABUSE
A Case Analysis for Health Care Providers

CYNTHIA SHELBY-LANE

I pushed her, I know I shouldn't have but I had a bad day and she knocked her false teeth off the shelf (Nurse's aide).
I don't want to go [into the nursing home] but my daughter says if I don't sell the house and give her the money she won't have anything to do with me any more (Elderly patient).

It is believed that one million elderly persons are battered, neglected, or exploited each year by family members or caretakers (Riffer, 1985). As the number of elderly persons in the United States continues to increase, geriatric abuse, which has become the most recent manifestation of domestic violence, is also likely to increase.

Maltreatment of the aged may be more difficult to identify than child abuse or spouse abuse for several reasons. Victims are reluctant to report abuse; many cases involve only subtle signs and have a great potential to pass undetected. In addition, there is relative isolation of the elderly abused person. Thus it is essential for providers to understand this and to focus on the many forms of elder abuse, since some are not always obvious and may not be detected as physical cruelty. Due to the demands placed upon physicians working in a busy emergency department, however, it is difficult to identify these victims of violence. This chapter will offer health providers some information about identifying geriatric abuse and will establish a protocol that can be used to detect and evaluate victims of this type of violence.

BACKGROUND OF THE PROBLEM

Elder abuse is not new, but recognition among the general public just began to surface in the 1980s. The 1960s were an era associated with recognizing child abuse. During the 1970s, we increasingly recognized spouse abuse. We began to recognize elder or geriatric abuse in the 1980s, and in the 1990s we may be able to deal with it effectively. Elder abuse is currently at the stage that child abuse was 20 years ago. Much less has been written about elder abuse. A great deal of public concern has been expressed in reference to the abuse of children and spouses but elder abuse essentially has been ignored, overlooked, and believed nonexistent.

Many of us would rather not think about the fact that the elderly among us are vulnerable—that in our community there are people who need protection from family members or even professional caregivers. What drives a person to violence against someone he or she loves or has loved—someone who trusts, or has trusted, him or her? Why does love turn to hate and neglect? What tensions exist within the family that such feelings of brutality are so near the surface? How can we as health care professionals be gentle and caring with our own mothers and grandmothers and then go to work and be impatient and careless with someone else's loved one?

Some of the reasons are related to the implications of aging America (Ansello, 1988). Old age is the most varied time in life. The elderly are a diverse group who are living longer than ever. A significant proportion of the elderly are women. A 50-year-old woman can expect to live an additional 31 years, and the life expectancy of a 75-year-old woman is an additional 12 years. Due to medical and technological advances, many older women, as well as their male counterparts, are living with disabling conditions. Their health and social needs have caught service systems off guard and unprepared. There is an inability of the federal and local governments to keep pace with the social and health care funding. In the past, nursing homes housed most of the disabled elderly of our society but, in general, the trend is away from institutionalization. The cost of such care is a factor since few can afford to be private pay patients in a nursing home. The nursing home industry also is shifting toward more acute rather than chronic care, and the residents of nursing homes look more like hospital residents 10 years ago, especially with the early discharge home from hospitals. Thus many older people are returning to their homes after spending time in nursing homes; others never enter these facilities in the first place but require care.

Parent caring is becoming an increasingly prevalent pattern. Providing such care, however, is a major source of stress to many children. It is believed to be a factor in elder abuse. Implications for caregiving, therefore, involve gerontological social workers, nursing programs, and a small number of physicians as well as physician groups.

MAGNITUDE OF THE PROBLEM

Elder abuse is, in essence, a hidden problem, so it is difficult to estimate the magnitude (Council on Scientific Affairs, 1987). It is hidden because older patients deny abuse has occurred, because health professionals cannot detect it, and because media coverage for this problem has been extremely scant.

Data documenting the extent of the problem have not been available until recently. Research on domestic violence focused primarily on child and spouse abuse, so few data were collected about the neglect and abuse of elderly persons by family members. This topic received little attention in the medical or nursing literature despite surveys that document exposure of professional caregivers to increasing numbers of elderly victims.

In 1980, the U.S. Senate Special Committee on Elder Abuse reported that 500,000 to 2.5 million cases of geriatric abuse, neglect, or mistreatment occur each year in this country. On the basis of its own survey, the U.S. House of Representatives Select Committee on Aging estimated that 4% of the nation's elderly population, or approximately 1 million persons, are victims of abuse. It appears that 1 out of every 25 persons older than 65 is abused, but only one 1 of every 5 persons who is a victim of elder abuse gets reported. This is in contrast to child abuse where 1 out of every 3 children who are abused gets reported.

Compounding the problem of determining the number of abused elders is the general lack of consensus on the definition of geriatric abuse and the ambiguity of many definitions used in state reporting law. In March of 1985, the Elder Abuse Prevention Identification and Treatment Act (HR 1674) was introduced in Congress. Among other provisions, this legislation served to clarify and standardize the language relating to geriatric abuse. Abuse, physical harm, exploitation, and neglect were defined.

In this work, the following categories and definitions of abuse will be used. Physical abuse is defined as willful direct infliction of physical pain or injury. It is the denial of physical and health-related necessities for the existence of life. Physical neglect includes the lack of attention, abandonment, and confinement of the elderly by family members or society. Psychological abuse and neglect is defined as the removal of the decision-making power from the elderly. It is the withholding of affection as well as social isolation. Material abuse/exploitation is any situation involving the dishonest use of an elderly person's resources, such as money or property. It is also misappropriation of health care resources. The violation of rights includes the denial of the basic rights of the aged person, which include having necessities such as food and decent housing, feeling useful and respected, having adequate medical care, and obtaining employment based on merit. The violation of rights also extends to isolating the victim from sharing in community recreational and educational resources, as well as having moral and financial support stripped from them. The elderly person is also limited with respect to access to knowledge on how to improve his or her life and is not able to find resources that enable fair improvement. It also deals with the issue of living and dying with dignity, which also may be taken away from or not afforded the victim.

OLDER PERSONS AT RISK FOR ABUSE

It is necessary to define the older, at-risk population before we can propose interventions or methods of prevention. The family is at the center of this identification process. Violent trends in American society have, in general, involved the family.

Several books have been written that show the family context of elder abuse. Strauss, Gelles, and Steinmetz (1980) found in their study of 2,143 families that 1 out of 8 couples showed trends of violence across three generations. So, do violent grandparents become victims? The study suggested that families who react to stress by behaving aggressively toward children and spouses are not likely to exclude the elderly, and, yes, grandparents do become victims of their own violence. Current statistics indicate that violence in the family is on the rise. Block and Sinnott (1979) looked at isolated versus chronic incidents of abuse. They found that there was a 58% incidence of previous episodes of abuse. This was an important finding clarifying whether abuse tends to occur repeatedly or as an isolated incident.

Additional studies also indicate that victims are chronically abused. Working with professionals in Massachusetts, O'Malley and associates showed that 70% of abuse cases were repetitive (O'Malley, Segars, Perez, Mitchela, & Kneupfel, 1979). Conditions that precipitate neglect and abuse seem to be chronic and ongoing, in general.

Who are the victims of elder abuse? No group is ever immune. The problem cuts across all social classes as well as all racial, ethnic, and religious groups. The typical victim profile is that of a Protestant, middle-class female, who is approximately 65 to 70 years of age, white, frail, mentally or physically impaired, dependent, and living with relatives. The victim usually resides in his or her own home or in the home of a close relative. This is an important distinction from the individual who has typically been thought to be the victim of elder abuse—the institutionalized person.

A person who needs care is at risk for abuse. A study by Pillemer and Wolf (1983) examined the role of dependency in abuse. They conducted a comparative study of 65 patients who were physically abused and 49 who were not, and found greater mental impairment in the abused group versus the unabused group. This impairment included recent dependency, depression, stubbornness, and isolation—which was a reaction to their dependency and the fact that the victim wanted to hold on to his past life of control. The fact that elder abuse crosses all social, economic, and ethnic backgrounds means that there is a trend toward disintegration of family balance.

THEORIES OF ELDER ABUSE

Causative theories for elder abuse are numerous and variable. They are not well understood but there is a strong correlation between dependency, disability, and abuse. Three models exist that attempt to explain the causation of elder abuse: the Psychopathological Model, the Learning Model, and the Situational Stress Model. The Psychopathological Model gives rise to the pathologic abuser who abuses substances such as drugs or alcohol, or who exhibits sociopathic behavior and may imitate acts of random violence. The Learning Model suggests that violence is passed on from generation to generation. It proposes that violent parents who abuse their children have children who become abusive parents and therefore incur the risk of abuse at an older age. The Situational Stress Model is based upon a stress "buildup" contention. The physically dependent elderly patient creates physical, mental, and financial stress for his or her caregiver. The caregiver becomes exhausted or antagonized, and this leads to violence as a result of his or her depression, hostility, and anger.

DETECTING ABUSE

What are the problems in detecting abuse? Physicians are in strategic positions to be able to identify abused elderly people (Cochran & Petrone, 1987; Council on Scientific Affairs, 1987; O'Brien, 1986). Yet this does not occur on a frequent and ongoing basis. Most studies show that the elderly suffer from neglect. This neglect includes psychological and physical abandonment, such as leaving the patient alone or tying him or her to a chair or bed for days. Physical findings include the breakdown of skin. Physical neglect, although rare, includes the withholding of food and medicine and, in some cases, actual beating of the victim.

In general, the problem of detecting abuse is related not only to the lack of definition but also to underreporting. The symptoms of aging seem to go unrecognized by professionals and the public and may lead to the lack of recognition of abuse or neglect. The issue of reporting is one that has not been addressed uniformly and justly by all states. Of the 41 states with laws that address adult victim abuse, only 21 states have a mandatory reporting law for victims aged 18 through 65, and only 17 states address the issue of elderly abuse. The person or agency required to report includes everything from human services agencies, courts, hospitals, nursing associations, and the general public. The general public, which is an anonymous group, generally reports about 20% of cases of abuse.

Recognition of suspicion of abuse is one of our biggest challenges, especially in the hospital emergency department. The patient will have medical complaints. The patient brought in by EMS, for instance, will have medical complaints whereby he is assessed with the usual history and physical. The physician may not always be in a position to see the patient's condition upon arrival and therefore may miss observing how the patient was dressed, or even detecting an unusual odor that might indicate neglect. The physical indicators must be addressed by the physician, and the physician must increase his or her observational skills suggesting that sometimes human tissue often can tell more than human lips. The patient may not be willing or even able to state that "I have been abused" or "I have been neglected." Behavior indicators also are a key factor in recognizing abuse in patients. They may be withdrawn or shy, and this may be mistaken for their usual personality as opposed to one that has been developed through victimization. Environmental indicators to look for are the caregiver's neglect to an obvious injury, a generalized fear on the part of the patient, the caregiver's obsession with control and with being present, and his or her lack of willingness to leave the patient's bedside.

Warning signs of abuse include bruises, welt cigarette burns, facial lacerations, and scalp bleeding (Fulmer, Street, & Carr, 1984; Jones, Dougherty, Schelble, & Cunningham, 1988). These are physical signs that should not be ignored and should obviate the need for further investigation. It is when these injuries are seen and recognized that further questioning of the patient and the caregivers should be done. The questioning should not be done in a hospital manner, but these types of injuries may be your only clue to the fact that the patient is a victim, is in a hostile environment, and may not be willing to say anything that may put his or her condition in further jeopardy. When the patient is a victim of psychological neglect or abuse, there is even more reluctance on the part of the victim to talk about the family and the conditions that exist at home. The victim may be extremely embarrassed by his or her situation, and this increases reluctance to seek help even when he or she knows that help is the only solution to the problem.

PERPETRATORS

Who is the perpetrator? The perpetrator of elder abuse most often is a relative of the victim and has taken care of that person for a number of years. The caretaker is burdened with stresses, which include financial demands, changes in life-style, and social isolation (Mildenberger & Wessman, 1986).

The abuser profile is one that shows that 75% of abusers are over 50 years of age, 20% over 70 years of age, and 40% are spouses of the victims. It is interesting to note that 50% of the abusers were children or grandchildren of the victim, and that the abuser usually was the least socially integrated in society and, therefore, had been delegated the caregiver responsibility due to lack of other responsibilities. The abuser profile also shows a family member in 80% to 96% of cases. Daughters perpetrate psychological abuse, whereas sons perpetrate physical abuse. In order of frequency, it is daughters and sons, then spouses, then grandchildren, siblings, nieces, nephews, and cousins who engage in abuse. Abusers often suffer from stress, drug addiction, chronic medical or financial problems, and alcoholism.

INTERVENTION

Multidimensional and multifactorial interventions are necessary that will require the assistance of numerous agencies in our society. The key is education and prevention, but intervention will have a major role as well

(Douglas, 1986; Phillips & Rempusheski, 1985). The overall goal is to benefit the abused elder. Forty percent of the elderly in one study refused intervention due to fear and embarrassment. A variety of local community agencies need to be involved to help improve the well-being of the abused and the abuser's ability to cope with the situation and obtain counseling. Hospital social workers represent a valuable resource with respect to intervention because, for the inexperienced and unknowledgeable physician, this is perhaps the only link with the possible solution to the problem (Goodwin, 1985). Adult protective services are extremely useful in trying to provide intervention for the victim of elder abuse. Out of 41 states, 21 had regulations for elder abuse linked with adult protective services in 1986. The legislation stated that to declare a person incompetent that person must (a) suffer from a long-term condition affecting their mental capacity, and (b) exhibit certain functional incapacities. Again, it must be recognized that many victims of elder abuse are reluctant to get involved in any legal action that involves adult protection services due to fear of retaliation. The knowledge that the caregiver may remove all care produces anxiety and, should the older person have to go back and live with the caregiver, he or she may perceive a "catch-22" situation with respect to initiating legal action. In some instances, victims might feel that they may be leaving a bad situation to go to a worse situation.

What can be done to help the elderly family caregiver adjust? An exploratory study concerning needs of caregivers found that, basically, the caregivers felt that there was a need for concrete services as well as financial resources and home health and assistance. Responses also suggested socialization needs of caregivers. They need to be educated about the caregiving role. An understanding of the needs of caregivers will help those professionals involved with providing solutions to this problem to develop programs that will be beneficial to society in general.

Physician education is critical. Residency programs need to develop a curriculum that addresses the issue of aging society and, in particular, the recognition of elder abuse.

The American Medical Association reported on diagnostic guidelines and treatment of elder abuse (Council on Scientific Affairs, 1987). Their findings concerning elder abuse and neglect helped develop model legislation for mandatory reporting by physicians for cases of elder abuse. (At present this is still not a mandated policy.)

We now recognize that the physician must investigate and understand family dynamics when confronting the abused, yet denying, elderly patient. Although adult protective services and programs exist in some areas, mandatory reporting does not. The legal backbone, therefore, is missing. There also is the problem of lack of federal policy on the issue of elder abuse and, in general, lack of uniform support from the federal government.

Prevention is the area where we probably can make our greatest strides. The Elder Abuse Prevention Identification and Treatment Act of 1985 (HR 1674), a complete study of the national incidence of elder abuse, was an effort addressed toward prevention. This law proposed a national printing house, codifying and standardizing the language relating to elder abuse, and funds to address the problem. The terminology of HR 1674 included the four terms *abuse, exploitation, neglect,* and *physical harm.* These terms still have not been incorporated into the uniform and general language of those persons who come in contact with victims of elder abuse.

Other efforts to prevent the problem of elder abuse are similar to those used to prevent child and spouse abuse. They include increased awareness, intervention procedures, and use of community resources.

As a physician who often treats older abused patients, I recommend that adult protective services become more involved in domestic situations and more concerned with dependent adults in intake households. In addition to adult protective services, I also would strongly recommend increased basic and continuing education for professional health care workers. These professionals are responsible for investigating charges of elder abuse, but often lack the advanced skills necessary to deal with the complex issues encountered. Also, public campaigns are needed to focus attention on the seriousness of elder abuse and to help raise the consciousness of all in our society regarding our personal responsibility for recognizing and reporting abuse.

As more people live longer, chronic diseases—most commonly conditions of middle and old age—have emerged as major causes of death and disability. There are now many more persons suffering from conditions that are managed or controlled rather than cured. Because these conditions often are of long duration, they create burdens for the individual and for society . Abuse is related to this. Elder abuse is, in many instances, the result of failure to provide a comprehensive continuum of care for the elderly, their families, and society as a whole. It is part of the largest social problem in contemporary American life—violence.

REFERENCES

Ansello, E. (1988). A view of aging America and some implications. *Caring,* 4-8.

Block, M. R., & Sinnott, J. D. (Eds.). (1979). *The battered elder syndrome.* College Park: University of Maryland, Center on Aging.

Cochran, C., & Petrone, S. (1987). Elder abuse: The physician's role in identification and prevention. *Illinois Medical Journal, 171,* 241-246.

Council on Scientific Affairs. (1987). Elder abuse and neglect. *Journal of the American Medical Association, 257*, 996-971.

Douglas, R. (1986). Domestic mistreatment of the elderly--Towards prevention. The Beth Israel Hospital Elder Assessment Team: An elder abuse assessment team in an acute hospital setting. *The Gerontologist, 26*, 115-118.

Fulmer, T., Street, S., & Carr, K. (1984). Abuse of the elderly: Screening and detection. *Journal of Emergency Nursing, 10*, 131-140.

Goodwin, J. (1985). Family violence: Principles of intervention and prevention. *Hospital and Community Psychiatry, 36*, 1074-1079.

Jones, J., Dougherty, J., Schelble, D., & Cunningham, W. (1988). Emergency department protocol for the diagnosis and evaluation of geriatric abuse. *Annals of Emergency Medicine, 17*, 1006-1015.

Mildenberger, C., & Wessman, H. (1986). Abuse and neglect of elderly persons by family members—A special communication. *Physical Therapy, 66*, 537-539.

O'Brien, J. (1986). Elder abuse and the physician. *Michigan Medicine, 85*, 618-620.

O'Malley, H., Segars, H., Perez, R., Mitchela, V., & Kneupfel, G. (1979). *Elder abuse in Massachusetts: A survey of professionals and paraprofessionals.* Boston: Legal Research and Services for the Elderly.

Phillips, L., & Rempusheski, V. (1985). A decision-making model for diagnosing and intervening in elder abuse and neglect. *Nursing Research, 34*, 134-139.

Pillemer, K. A., & Wolf, R. S. (1983). *Organizational assessment of the delivery of protective services to abused and neglected elders at two home care corporations.* Worcester: University of Massachusetts Medical Center, Center on Aging.

Riffer, J. (1985). Elder abuse victims estimated at 1 million. *Hospitals, 57*, 60.

Strauss, M. A., Gelles, R. J., & Steinmetz, S. K. (1980). *Behind closed doors: Violence in the American family.* Garden City, NY: Anchor.

Chapter 7

HEALTH, POLICY, AND AGED MINORITIES

JOHN B. WALLER, JR.

One of the greatest public health and public policy challenges today is how to shape a reasonable, dignified, affordable, and humane long-term care policy. The black elderly share with the white elderly many problems, both medical and social. However, a number of specific characteristics affecting the black elderly exacerbate and circumscribe their medical and social problems in ways different from the white elderly and, indeed, in some instances, different from most other minorities. Sensitivity to both the similarities and the differences between the black, other minority, and white elderly is crucial to the formulation of humane, cost-effective public policy designed to meet the challenges to the provision of health care to the minority elderly and generally improve their poorer health status.

Whenever the subject of health care for the elderly is discussed there is a natural tendency to focus on the Medicare system as if it were a near adequate governmental response to long-term care needs. In fact, especially problematic are the many services Medicare does not cover, such as preventive checkups, outpatient medication, and institutional long-term care. Neither does it provide for in-home care with the exception of minimal coverage for speech therapy, occupational therapy, and social work services. Furthermore, with an increasing out-of-pocket share of health care costs borne by the older person, Medicare is not well suited for the health problems of an older population. The 23 million Americans older than 65 represent 11% of our population, yet they account for over half of the more than $40 billion federal health care budget and almost 30% of the total of $160 billion spent each year on health care in this country. This 11% of the population occupies approximately 33% of all nursing home beds and consumes over 25% of all prescription drugs. The per capita expenditures of the aged for all types of services exceeds that of all other segments of the population. Despite the large public investment in their health expenses, the elderly still pay a substantial and increasing portion of their health care bill out of what is most often a limited, fixed income (Ouslander & Beck, 1982), and their need for long-term care is escalating.

Long-term care presents problems of quality, access, and cost. Quality services should be reasonably accessible to those in need without regard to financial or other barriers; the costs must be affordable by individuals and society. The long-term care problem in the United States is not simply how our society can afford to care for all elderly and dependent persons from available public and private dollars; the problem is how to develop an acceptable system with less of a physical, financial, emotional, and social toll on elderly citizens and their families when they need care. It is a problem that is very salient to the health of the aged and particularly critical for older minorities.

This chapter focuses primarily on the black elderly because, despite the problems mentioned above, there is more published data on the black elderly than on any other minority. This in no way should imply that there are not significant medical and social problems among the Hispanic, the Native American, the Asian Pacific Islanders, and the Arab elderly; nor is the challenge to find solutions to those problems through intelligent public policy any less important or acute. The black elderly population, those aged 65 and over, is growing more rapidly than the white elderly population. There are an estimated two million black elderly in this country, representing 9% of the estimated total 22 million elderly population (Siegel & Taeuber, 1986). As Gibson and Jackson (1987) point out, the disproportionate growth of the older black population is of social policy significance for several reasons. First, larger numbers of older blacks with chronic, physically limiting illnesses will further complicate payment of the health care bills of an aging population (Davis, 1986; Rice & Estes, 1984). Extraordinary strains will be placed on already burdened black families, and long-term care policies for an aging society need careful development (Soldo & Manton, 1985). The debate, thus far, has not considered the interplay among the special life circumstances of blacks and other ethnic minorities. It has not considered their levels of physical functioning, their traditional and current patterns of informal support, and their health care needs.

Consider briefly some demographic statistics of note, especially those factors that influence the health of the elderly, their utilization of health services, and their contributions to health care expenditures. Life expectancy has increased dramatically in the United States in this century, rising from 47.3 years in 1900 to 72 years and 79 years for white men and women, respectively, in 1983. This contrasts with a life expectancy of 65 years for black men and 74 years for black women in that same year, a gap of 5.6 years between black and white figures. Although the 5.6-year disparity in life expectancy may not seem that significant, blacks today have a life expectancy already reached by whites in the early 1950s, or a lag of about 40 years.

Although the overall life expectancy may not increase substantially through the early 1990s, the number of persons surviving to old age will increase. This is important because illness and disability increases with advancing age, especially so for those older than 75 who comprise the most rapidly growing segment of the elderly population. Life expectancy at birth is less for blacks than whites, largely due to the higher rate of infant deaths and the vastly higher death rate for young black men. For those persons who do reach age 65, however, the life expectancy for blacks and whites is much closer. Aged blacks have lower death rates for many diseases than do whites. This "survivor effect" has been attributed to hardiness among survivors in a population that has experienced a high early-age death rate (Jackson, 1980; Markides & Mindel, 1987; U.S. Department of Health and Human Services, 1985). In the city of Detroit, the elderly comprise nearly 12% of the population compared to 11% nationwide. Life expectancy at age 65 for black males in Detroit is higher than the nationwide average for black males (13.9 versus 13.3 years) and is higher than that of white males in Detroit (13.4 at age 65).

The geographic distribution of ethnic minority populations is another important demographic consideration. With the exception of the American Indians, most ethnic minority groups in the United States are highly urbanized, even more so than the dominant white population. According to the 1980s United States census, 80.6% of black elderly live in urban areas compared to 73.8% of the white elderly. Among the three subpopulations of black, Hispanic, and white, blacks are more likely to reside in central cities although Hispanics are actually the most urbanized overall of these groups.

While primarily urban, whites are twice as likely to be found outside the central cities as within. American Indians remain largely rural, although this may result in part from inadequate enumeration of urban Indians.

Two other important demographic factors that influence the health status of the elderly are income and living arrangements. Minority aged have always had a much lower standard of living than white aged. In spite of the fact that the percentage of elderly falling below the poverty level has declined for a number of years, the number of minority elderly in poverty is still substantially greater than the number of elderly in the majority white group. The percentage of the elderly in poverty, in both black and white groups, has declined dramatically since 1959. In 1983, only 12% of the white elderly were in poverty compared to almost three times as many blacks (36.3%) and twice as many Hispanic elderly (23.1%).

The cost of living is rising faster for the elderly than for the rest of the population. This faster rise in the senior price index is attributed to greater elderly spending than the general population on medical care and shelter items that have increased rapidly in cost from 1982 to 1987. The relatively high levels of poverty among blacks and some of the other ethnic minority groups can be attributed in part to low levels of education. It is not surprising that the level of education of white elderly is considerably higher than that of blacks or Hispanics, both for males and females. The disparities are much greater for females than for males. Since level of education is an important predictor of earning power, the consequences of this can be quite severe in old age.

It is now a well-known fact that there has been a growing disparity between the numbers of elderly males and elderly females. The health status of elderly women is of particular concern due to a number of social and demographic factors. Elderly females currently outnumber elderly males by 1.48 to 1. With the expanding gap in life expectancy (77.5 for females versus 70.0 for males in 1980), this ratio will increase significantly. Elderly females are much more likely to be widowed and living alone than elderly males and thus are more likely to suffer from the social isolation that is known to be a risk factor for premature dependency (Unpublished testimony, 1986). As the gap in life expectancy for black females and males widens (and it is already wider than the gap between white females and males), the jeopardy of greater social isolation and the risk of dependency among aged black women will be increased substantially. Combined with the excess of poverty among the black elderly, these data only confirm the need for a special public health policy on the needs of elderly black women.

Despite the many serious problems facing black communities and their elderly residents, a growing body of research statistics indicate that the black aged are more integrated into their environment and are generally less isolated than the white elderly. It is this strong network of social support for the aged in the black community that must be kept in mind and built upon by public policy initiatives designed to improve the health status of the black elderly. Gibson and Jackson (1987) point out that the quality and quantity of informal support available to the black elderly will have profound effects on their need for long-term care. They further point out that a small but growing body of literature suggests that the informal support for older blacks—help from friends, family, and church—is important to their physical health and effective functioning and that exchanges within the social networks of older blacks have some insulation qualities.

The social epidemiological literature also emphasizes the importance of informal support in health and functioning. Social ties affect the etiology and course of disease, physical functioning, and even mortality. Further, it has been determined that the friend and kin networks of blacks generally expand rather than contract in successively older age groups. The oldest old's helpers are more varied, but the majority of the black elderly receive help in the form of goods and services from family members, emotional support in form of advice, counsel, encouragement, moral support, validation of attitudes and perceptions from friends, and prayer from church members. The challenge to evolving long-term care public policy is to build upon these strengths rather than force disruptions in these social networks through ill-conceived rules, regulations, and eligibility requirements for publicly funded programs.

As I explore further those factors that are shaping the challenges to providing health care to the black and minority elderly, some health status indicators need to be examined. Measurement of the health status of the elderly relies upon data concerning both mortality and morbidity. Although mortality data are valuable, they tell little or nothing about the prevalence of nonfatal conditions such as arthritis, sensory impairment, and organic brain syndrome that are known to be particular burdens of the aged. Despite this limitation, mortality data do have advantages because they are routinely collected for all persons from death certificates. Information regarding morbidity, or illness, on the other hand, is collected from various national surveys and does not include information on all individuals. Thus in this presentation I will attempt to compare mortality rates for the city of Detroit to those of the United States. I can provide only national data regarding the prevalence of various nonfatal, but potentially disabling, conditions.

Mortality trends reveal that enormous progress has been made in the past 40 years in reducing death rates among all aged Americans, with the reduction being twice as great for females than for males from 1940 to 1978. Although improvement in survival was seen for each subgroup of the elderly during each of the four decades since 1940, the greatest reduction in death rates was enjoyed in the years 1969 to 1978 for men aged 65 to 69 and in persons of both sexes age 85 and older. Elderly blacks enjoyed substantial reductions in their death rates during this period as well, but significant gaps remain between death rates for elderly blacks and those for whites.

For both blacks and whites, heart disease, cancer, and cerebrovascular disease (stroke) have remained the three leading causes of death since 1950, and together they continue to account for 3 out of every 4 deaths among the population 65 years of age and older (see Satariano, Albert, & Belle, 1982, and Table 7.1). Because the known and suspected risk factors for cardiovascular and cerebrovascular disease are similar, I will discuss them together; this is followed by a discussion of the impact of cancer on the black elderly and a few points on deaths from diabetes mellitus and influenza infection.

Taken together, heart disease and stroke cause more deaths, disability, and economic loss in the United States than any other acute or chronic disease and are the leading causes of days lost from work for both blacks and whites (U.S. Department of Health and Human Services, 1985). Heart disease has remained the leading cause of death in the elderly since 1950. Among those 65 years and older, 44 of every 100 deaths in 1978 resulted from heart disease. Women have experienced more substantial reductions in death rates from heart disease than men in the last 35 years.

Significant differences exist between blacks and whites in the prevalence of various cardiovascular disease (CVD) risk factors. The principal treatable risk factors for CVD among whites include hypertension, elevated blood cholesterol, cigarette smoking, diabetes mellitus, and obesity. Although it has not been demonstrated conclusively by research, the data indicate that these same factors increase the risk of blacks for heart disease. Coronary heart disease mortality rates are similar in white and black men but are greater in black women than in white women. The number of new cases of coronary heart disease also may be increasing in black women compared to white women; however, some data indicate that the prevalence may be similar between black and whites of the same sex. Hospital admission records suggest higher rates of sudden death prior to hospital admission among black men (U.S. Department of Health and Human Services, 1985).

Stroke deaths are much more common among blacks than whites and a greater proportion of blacks than whites suffers nonfatal strokes. Also more common in blacks is end-stage renal disease, or kidney failure, which results

Table 7.1

Leading Causes of Death

Detroit and the United States, 1980

Ages 65 and Over

Cause	*Deaths per 100,000 Population*				
	All Races Male and Female	*Black Male*	*Black Female*	*White Male*	*White Female*
All Causes					
United States	5,251.9	6,935.6	4,775.3	6,444.4	4,522.5
Detroit	5,828.1	6,565.4	4,450.3	7,956.0	5,165.9
Diseases of heart					
United States	2,330.4	2,629.8	2,039.4	2,842.0	2,058.1
Detroit	2,805.5	2,722.2	2,090.0	3,855.5	2,719.4
Malignant neoplasms					
United States	1,011.3	1,646.8	782.1	1,369.8	777.5
Detroit	1,071.1	1,597.2	719.9	1,538.5	772.0
Cerebrovascular disease					
United States	573.1	722.0	655.8	550.6	585.6
Detroit	592.8	537.9	601.5	676.2	580.6
Pneumonia and influenza					
United States	178.1	216.2	116.6	214.6	160.3
Detroit	182.9	254.6	136.7	257.4	134.4
Chronic obstructive lung disease					
United States	170.6	174.1	37.8	315.2	90.0
Detroit	153.0	172.4	42.5	353.6	89.6
Diabetes mellitus					
United States	98.7	130.4	183.8	90.6	96.4
Detroit	117.4	90.3	161.0	114.8	105.9
Accidents and adverse effects					
United States	74.6	131.0	84.0	87.8	63.0
Detroit	86.1	131.4	39.5	133.4	67.2
Nephritis nephrotic syndrome and nephrosis					
United States	50.8	123.8	89.8	59.0	38.2
Detroit	74.7	110.9	100.2	74.4	42.8
Chronic liver disease and cirrhosis					
United States	37.3	48.2	21.8	57.5	25.1
Detroit	66.9	102.6	15.2	130.3	44.8
Homicide and legal intervention					
United States	5.5	31.2	8.1	6.8	2.9
Detroit	23.5	73.9	6.1	27.9	8.1
Suicide					
United States	17.8	11.5	1.5	37.9	6.5
Detroit	10.0	8.2	3.0	21.7	8.1

SOURCE: Unpublished testimony delivered to the United States House of Representatives Select Committee on Aging (1986, March 21). Presented by Stephen B. Blount, M.D., of the City of Detroit Health Department.

from hypertension. Not only are blacks more likely to develop high blood pressure, black hypertensives are at much greater risk for end-stage renal disease than whites. Stroke mortality declined 51% and coronary heart disease declined 42% in blacks from 1968 to 1982. Hypertension control contributed much to this success, but significant excess morbidity and mortality is still suffered by blacks from high blood pressure. In terms of risk factors, cigarette smoking is more prevalent among blacks than whites, as is diabetes mellitus (diagnosed and undiagnosed) and obesity among black women. Each of these factors is in some way amenable to individual action and thus speak to the need for cost-effective health education programs among blacks.

Cancer is the second leading cause of death among adults in the United States, including those age 65 and over, and accounts for approximately 20% of all deaths among the elderly. The risk of developing cancer increases with age; 56% of all cancers are diagnosed among persons 65 years and older. The multiple and complex health problems faced by the aged serve to complicate the prevention, diagnosis, and treatment of cancer and increase their cancer burden, which is particularly heavy for the black elderly.

When one compares the rankings of cancer sites in incidence rates (that is the new case rates) for metropolitan Detroit white and black women and men aged 65 to 74 years old, for the years 1973 to 1982 (see Tables 7.2 and 7.3), one finds that although black and white women share the same three leading sites, important differences in rates exist between groups for these and other cancer sites. While elderly white women have a higher incidence rate than elderly black women for breast cancer, their death rates are quite similar. This fact, combined with the fact that the average size of a breast tumor at diagnosis is greater in black women than white, suggests that elderly black women breast cancer patients are diagnosed later and die in disproportionate numbers compared to whites for this most common site of cancer among women. Larger tumors at diagnosis are less amenable to treatment and require more disfiguring surgery, which has devastating effects on both self-image and prospects for employment. Incidence rates among elderly black women are higher for the two most common cancer sites among all aged women—the colon, and lung and bronchus.

Significantly, the incidence rate for invasive cervical cancer is almost 2 1/2 times greater among elderly black women than among elderly white women. This is notable because for a relatively long time, there has been a reliable, noninvasive, and cost-effective method to screen women for cervical disease, the pap smear.

Table 7.2

A Ranking of Cancer Sites by Incidence Rates (per 100,000) for White and Black Females Aged 65 to 74 Years in the Detroit Metropolitan Area, 1973-1982.

| | *White* | | | *Black* | |
Rank	Site	Rate	Rank	Site	Rate
1	Breast	301.88	1	Breast	224.92
2	Colon	155.54	2	Colon	161.82
3	Lung and Bronchus	124.15	3	Lung and Bronchus	127.11
4	Corpus	109.39	4	Cervix	64.91
5	Ovary	50.51	5	Corpus	63.55
6	Ill-defined	44.11	6	Pancreas	60.85
7	Non-Hodgkin's Lymphoma	41.23	7	Ill-defined	48.68
8	Pancreas	39.37	8	Stomach	44.17
9	Rectum	37.61	9	Ovary	36.06
10	Urinary bladder	36.21	10	Multiple myeloma	31.55
11	Leukemia	29.90	11.5	Rectum	31.10
12	Stomach	27.67	11.5	Leukemia	31.10
13	Cervix	26.93	13	Urinary bladder	29.30
14	Head and Neck	21.91	14	Non-Hodgkin's	26.14
15	Kidney	21.36	15	Kidney	20.28
16	Multiple myeloma	18.76	16	Head and neck	18.03
17	Brain	14.95	17	Esophagus	15.23
18	Melanoma	10.59	18	Thyroid	8.11
19	Thyroid	9.01	19	Brain	6.31
20	Esophagus	8.26	20	Hodgkin's disease	3.16
21	Hodgkin's disease	3.99	21	Melanoma	2.25

SOURCE: Metropolitan Detroit Cancer Surveillance System, Division of Epidemiology, Michigan Cancer Foundation.

Unfortunately, many physicians discontinue routine cervical cancer examinations after the menopause when the risk of disease is actually greatest. Studies indicate that elderly black women are less likely than their white counterparts to have had a cervical examination (National Center for Health Statistics [NCHS], 1981). Black women age 65 and older in metropolitan Detroit also experience higher incidence rates than elderly white women in the metropolitan Detroit area for cancers of pancreas, stomach, and esophagus, and for multiple myeloma.

Black men aged 65 to 74 years in metropolitan Detroit have higher incidence rates than white men of similar age for cancers of the prostate, lung and bronchus, stomach, and pancreas, and for multiple myeloma (see Table 7.3). Death rates for these and other cancer sites, particularly the colon,

Table 7.3

A Ranking of Cancer Sites by Incidence Rates (per 100,000) for White and Black Males Aged 65 to 74 Years in the Detroit Metropolitan Area, 1973-1982.

| | *White* | | | *Black* | |
Rank	*Site*	*Rate*	*Rank*	*Site*	*Rate*
1	Lung and bronchus	508.89	1	Prostate	700.22
2	Prostate	400.45	2	Lung and bronchus	606.42
3	Colon	210.14	3	Colon	189.26
4	Urinary bladder	164.35	4	Stomach	99.87
5	Rectum	78.49	5	Urinary bladder	79.46
6	Head and neck	72.63	6	Esophagus	72.84
7	Stomach	71.38	7	Pancreas	72.28
8	Ill-defined	63.39	8	Ill-defined	67.32
9	Pancreas	59.40	9	Head and neck	59.04
10	Leukemia	55.41	10	Rectum	57.24
11	Larynx	53.16	11	Larynx	49.66
12	Non-Hodgkin's lymphoma	48.54	12	Multiple myeloma	45.25
13	Kidney	46.67	13	Leukemia	44.70
14	Esophagus	34.44	14	Kidney	35.31
15	Brain	24.46	15	Non-Hodgkin's disease	3.86
16	Multiple myeloma	21.34	16	Brain	7.73
17	Melanoma	19.72	17	Hodgkin's disease	3.86
18	Hodgkin's disease	7.36	18	Melanoma	3.31
19	Thyroid	5.24	19	Thyroid	2.21
20	Testes	1.00	20	Testes	0.55

SOURCE: Metropolitan Detroit Cancer Surveillance System, Division of Epidemiology, Michigan Cancer Foundation

and the head and neck, are also higher in aged black men, perhaps resulting from later diagnosis. The fact that many of the cancer sites where incidence and mortality is high for blacks also are sites where in the use of both tobacco and alcohol are risk factors suggests that individual and societal, including governmental, actions must be taken to prevent cancer and promote health.

Death resulting from pneumonia and influenza comprise the fourth largest number of deaths among the aged in the United States. Death rates among Detroit's elderly for pneumonia and influenza increased between 1980 to 1984. This is noteworthy because of the availability of a safe, reliable, and cost-effective vaccine against influenza infection. Community-based immunizations programs targeted toward seniors can have a substantial impact in reducing preventable deaths from pneumonia and influenza. Finally, mortality rates in Detroit for diabetes mellitus are significantly higher among black women age 65 and over than among elderly white women. Combined with obesity, which is more common among black women than white, diabetes mellitus produces substantially higher risks for other chronic conditions. Diabetes is a risk factor for coronary heart disease and peripheral vascular disease, and its complications include kidney failure, eye disease, and vascular complications that may result in amputations (U.S. Department of Health and Human Services, 1985).

A brief look at morbidity estimates will show that the most frequent nonfatal, chronic conditions and impairments for older people are arthritis, which affects 44%, and high blood pressure, which affects 35%. Reduced vision affects 22%; impaired hearing, 29%; and heart condition, 20%. The prevalence of nutritional deficiencies, depression associated with social isolation, and mental disorientation is not known, but when elderly persons are confronted with combinations of these often competing problems over time, their ability to cope with them can be so eroded that they decline into dependency. The major challenge to prevention in the elderly is to intervene effectively at various points in the natural histories of the conditions and at sufficiently early stages to intercept and/or retard this process. The following have been identified as physical and social risk factors for premature dependency: (a) social isolation; (b) uncorrected sensory impairment; (c) poor nutrition; and (d) over-medication (Branch & Jette, 1982; National Institute on Aging, 1985).

Although older blacks suffer less social isolation than elderly whites (NCHS, 1984), they may have a higher prevalence rate than their white counterparts for the other risk factors for premature dependency. Blacks more often than whites suffer from uncorrected visual impairment, and this perhaps holds true for hearing impairment as well (NCHS, 1984). Poor nutrition contributes to the obesity that is more common among older black women than whites. The lower average level of education among older blacks increases their risk of overmedication as it limits their ability to understand and comply with the often complicated therapeutic regimens for their more common multiple conditions. Two of the principle measures of morbidity are the number of days of bed disability and hospital days. Blacks in general, and elderly blacks in particular, consistently report higher rates for both of these measures than do their white counterparts (NCHS, 1981; NCHS, 1984).

Despite the strength they derive from being more socially supported and less isolated than elderly white women, older black women share a health status profile that remains quite tragic; this is largely due to their greater poverty. As noted earlier, elderly black women in metropolitan Detroit have higher incidence rates than elderly white women for cancers of the colon, lung and bronchus, pancreas, esophagus, stomach, and for multiple myeloma (see Table 7.2). Older black women have high blood pressure significantly more often than older white women, resulting in higher reported prevalence of hypertensive heart disease, diabetes, and stroke. Diabetes among aged black women contributes to the situation in which they more often than elderly white women suffer from visual impairment and hypertension. Obesity, also more common among elderly black women, is a risk factor for hypertension and diabetes.

Finally, uncorrected sensory impairment, noted above as a risk factor for premature dependency in the elderly, exacts a high cost from elderly black women in terms of overall quality of life. The need for eye treatment among black adults was found to be significantly higher than that for whites (NCHS, 1983). The greater poverty among elderly black women provides a significant barrier to their receiving treatment for both visual and hearing impairment.

The health care utilization patterns of elderly black women provide another lens through which the particular social and medical disadvantages of this population can be viewed. Ambulatory care visits to physician offices are less frequent among aged black women than white. The excess incidence of invasive cervical cancer among black women (see Table 7.2) clearly suggests that preventive care, including routine cervical cancer screening with a pelvic examination and pap smear, is not being made sufficiently available and/or is not being used. Mortality rates and age-specific incidence rates for cervical cancer both increase with age, indicating both the need and the opportunity for aggressive screening among the elderly black female population, which is at higher risk than older white females for invasive cervical neoplasm (Satariano, Albert, & Belle, 1982).

No discussion of health status of the black aged can be meaningful without a special focus on the health problems of the elderly black woman, who more often survives to old age and thus is subject to greater risk of disease and need for services. In 1980, there were 148 women age 65 and over for every 100 men of the same age in the United States. The 7-year difference in life expectancy by sex among all Americans (which accounted for the greater number of females in 1980) is expected to increase to a 10-year difference by the year 2003. If this trend holds for the black elderly as well, and the already wider gap between black male and female life expectancy continues to expand, the problems of the black aged will be largely the problems faced by older black women.

Elderly black women have fewer financial resources to draw upon than white women of the same age and thus are at a particular disadvantage when confronted with major health problems. Among all women age 65 and over, 41% of black women have incomes below the poverty level, compared to

15% of white women. Among elderly women living with families, 6% of white women had incomes below the poverty level compared to 29% of black women. The poverty of black women is accentuated if they do not live with families or if they maintain a family without a husband (21% for black women compared to 8% for white women). Elderly black women are nearly three times as likely as white women to be recipients of public assistance.

The distinguishing feature of the health status of elderly women is the greater prevalence of chronic illnesses that cause limitations in how they live, and these illnesses often are multiple. Women have higher rates of long-term chronic diseases, while men have higher rates of fatal diseases. According to national surveys, women report a higher incidence than men of hypertension, arthritis, diabetes, anemia, thyroid disorders, urinary tract disease, chronic sinusitis, gallbladder disease, and numerous gastrointestinal conditions and orthopedic impairments.

The rate of hospital use is lower for elderly black women than for their white counterparts. This has been attributed to a greater tendency of black women than of white women to delay treatment until later stages of disease. Blacks have been found to visit physicians for mandatory, as compared to elective, care more often than whites, and they have also been found to receive fewer preventive services than whites (NCHS, 1984). The lower rate of hospital use by elderly black women cannot be surprising and only serves to increase their burden when ill. The higher hospital fatality rate among elderly black women compared to similar age white women may indicate that the conditions for which older black women enter hospitals are more serious and are perhaps at later stages of illness than they are for white women. (Satariano, Albert, & Belle). Fewer elderly black than white women reside in nursing homes (36 per 1,000 population compared to 62 per 1,000 population); the greater social integration enjoyed by blacks and their tendency to be less isolated contribute to this. Older black women are more likely to maintain an extended family household and thus have informal care available to them as a preferred alternative to institutionalization. Because of the greater poverty of older black women, their use of Medicaid as a source of payment for nursing home care limits their potential for nursing home care even when it is desired, because of the shortage of beds funded by Medicaid. In summary, the older black woman suffers from greater poverty than her white counterpart and has higher mortality and morbidity rates for such chronic conditions as high blood pressure, diabetes, visual impairments, and certain forms of cancer; she also reaps fewer benefits from the organized health care system. In spite of this, she generally is less socially isolated than her white counterpart and enjoys more support from her family and community; this support is critical to maintaining her autonomy and preventing her decline into dependency.

Addressing the special needs of the older black woman requires a focus on both the expansion of direct services and the financing mechanism to provide for them. The lower utilization of preventive services by elderly black women must be addressed by expanding health education and treatment services for the chronic conditions that most often affect them. Nutritional counseling, for example, can impact upon morbidity resulting from diabetes, hypertension, and obesity. The problems of overmedication can be addressed by helping the aged to manage their medications, as has been shown in demonstration projects. Financial barriers to screening, diagnosis, treatment, and extended care for cancers of the breast, colon, and cervix should be reduced. Medicare and Medicaid reimbursement rates for correction of visual and hearing impairments should be increased to the level prevailing in the private sector. Finally, in order to ensure that safe and reliable influenza vaccines are available at low cost, the federal government should explore mechanisms to limit the potential liability of vaccine manufacturers from lawsuits resulting from rare adverse immunization effects and/or explore the feasibility of governmental production of such vaccines.

Governmental action in terms of health care financing will be critical to efforts to improve the health status of black females over the age of 65. Reimbursement rates under Medicare and Medicaid should be made equal to rates prevailing in the private sector. An analysis of the extent to which co-payments are required from recipients for certain services, particularly screening, should be conducted. Those co-payments found to be barriers to care for patients unable to meet them should be eliminated. Elimination of these and other financial obstacles to care will reduce some of the delays in hospitalization disproportionately experienced by elderly black women. Home care alternatives to institutionalization should be encouraged through the provision of tax incentives to families and other significant informal providers of care to the elderly. For those who are poor and require institutionalization, more nursing home beds should be supported through the federal contribution to state-run Medicaid programs.

RECOMMENDATIONS

In summary, the picture of the health status of the black aged painted by the discussion above is an overwhelmingly bleak one, relieved only to a slight degree by the presence of greater social support for them through family and community members. A public health policy directed toward improving the health status of the black and other minority elderly, informed by meaningful analysis of relevant data and underlined by a humane and egalitarian approach to health care in the world's richest society, should consider the following recommendations that involve both health care financing and the delivery of direct services.

(1) Reduce financial barriers to care. Co-payments required by Medicare or Medicaid that are found to reduce or delay care for preventive and curative services should be eliminated.

(2) Encourage the development of home care alternatives to institutionalization. Demonstration projects that build upon existing informal networks that provide home care for older blacks should be established and rigorously evaluated with a view toward dissemination of cost-effective methods.

(3) Expand the provision of preventive health services. Health education services, including nutrition counseling, should be increased and focused on reducing risk factors for premature dependency among elderly populations, such as older blacks, who have a greater prevalence of these factors.

(4) Establish demonstration projects that assist the elderly in management of their medications. Federally funded, community-based programs that focus on the poorly educated older black and other minority persons are needed to reduce the morbidity from overmedication, which is largely preventable.

(5) Consider legislation to limit the legal liability of vaccine manufacturers and/or explore federal production of vaccines. The availability of safe, reliable, and cost-effective vaccines against influenza may be jeopardized if manufacturers conclude that the costs of defense against lawsuits resulting from alleged adverse immunization effects outweigh the relatively small profits derived from vaccine production.

(6) Consider legislation to end the federal subsidies to tobacco growers. The leading preventable cause of death in the United States is cigarette smoking, which increases the risk of contracting a number of the chronic diseases that affect the elderly and have their origins in the earlier adult years.

(7) Fund additional research on the health status of the black elderly. Despite the serious and widespread social and medical problems facing the black elderly, particularly older black women, relatively little research has been conducted looking at their particular characteristics and problems. Public health policy only can be as good as the data upon which it is based.

In my opinion, each recommendation is oriented toward maintaining functional autonomy among the elderly and preventing their slide into dependency. This is the major challenge to the provision of health care to black and other minority elderly.

REFERENCES

Branch, L. G., & Jette, A. M. (1982). A prospective study of long-term care institutionalization among the aged. *American Journal of Public Health, 72,* 1373-1379.

Davis, K. (1986). Aging and the heath-care system: Economic and structural issues. *Daedalus, 115,* 227-246.

Gibson, R. C., & Jackson, J. S. (1987). The health, physical functioning, and informal support of the black elderly. *The Milbank Quarterly, 65*(2), 421-454.

Jackson, J. J. (1980). *Minorities and aging.* Belmont, CA: Wadsworth.

Markides, K. S., & Mindel, C. H. (1987). *Aging and ethnicity.* Newbury Park, CA: Sage.

National Center for Health Statistics. (1980). *Health, United States, 1980* (DHHS Publication No. PHS 81-1232). Washington, DC: Government Printing Office.

National Center for Health Statistics. (1981, August). *Use of health services by women 65 years of age and over—United States*(DHHS Publication No. PHS 81-1720). Washington, DC: Government Printing Office.

National Center for Health Statistics. (1981, December). *Health, United States, 1981* (DHHS Publication No. PHS 82-1232). Washington, DC: Government Printing Office.

National Center for Health Statistics. (1983, March). *Eye conditions and related need for medical care among persons 1-74 years of age: United States, 1971-72* (DHHS Publication No. PHS 83-1678). Washington, DC: Government Printing Office.

National Center for Health Statistics. (1984). *Health indicators for Hispanic, black, and white Americans* (DHHS Publication No. 84-1576). Washington, DC: Government Printing Office.

National Institute on Aging. (1985). *Seventh report to council on program, October, 1985.* Washington, DC: Government Printing Office.

Ouslander, J. G., & Beck, J. C. (1982). Defining the health problems of the elderly. *Annual Review of Public Health, 3,* 55-83.

Rice, D. P., & Estes, C. L. (1984). Health of the elderly: Policy issues and challenges. *Health Affairs, 3,* 25-49.

Satariano, W. A., Albert, S., & Belle, S. H. (1982). Age and cancer incidence: A test of double jeopardy. *Journal of Gerontology, 37,* 642-647.

Siegel, J. S., & Taeuber, C. M. (1986). Demographic perspectives on the long-lived society. *Daedalus, 115,* 77-118.

Soldo, B. J., & Manton, K. G. (1985). Changes in the health status and service needs of the oldest old: Current patterns and future trends. *The Milbank Quarterly/Health and Society, 63*(2), 289-319.

U. S. Department of Health and Human Services. (1985). *Report of the Secretary's Task Force on Black and Minority Health, Vol. 1: Executive summary.* Washington, DC: Government Printing Office.

Unpublished testimony delivered to the United States House of Representatives Select Committee on Aging (1986, March 21). Presented by Stephen B. Blount, M.D., of the City of Detroit Health Department.

Part III

HEALTH PROBLEMS AND FAMILY CARE: IMPACT BEYOND THE OLDER PATIENT

Chapter 8

FAMILY CAREGIVING AS AN INTERGENERATIONAL TRANSFER

BARBARA HIRSHORN

Over the last several decades, an increasing proportion of Americans have survived to reach old age—particularly advanced old age. At the same time, caregiving as a resource that is transferred intergenerationally *within* the family has changed in emphasis and grown in importance as a center of attention for those who are concerned with the family context of older people. This chapter focuses upon some of the issues requiring close examination as a result of this change in emphasis and growth in importance. The discussion that follows will (a) illustrate how family caregiving occurs on both an everyday basis and on an extraordinary basis—and as a process that occurs across the life course; (b) describe some of the costs of family caregiving; and (c) discuss motivations for caregiving in terms of intergenerational aspects of family life.

CONCEPTUALIZING THE TRANSFER OF
CARE IN THE FAMILY CONTEXT

The various kinds of caregiving that occur within the context of the family are manifestations of a private intergenerational transfer that is universal and that exemplifies the strong bonds between generations. These intergenerational exchanges are so common and natural in the lives of those who live with or near blood relations or fictive kin that they often are not even recognized or acknowledged until and unless they cease for some reason (Kingson, Hirshorn, & Cornman, 1986).

Across cultures, it is clear that, from birth onward, most individuals will both receive care from and give care to family members—unless some seriously intrusive event or great disability impedes them from serving as caregivers. In this care exchange process family members share a great variety of resources intergenerationally (e.g., time, money, emotional support) (Kingson et al., 1986). These exchanges occur both between individuals who belong to the same generation—for example, sister to brother—and between individuals of different generations—for instance, daughter-in-law to mother-in-law.

There rarely is a one-to-one reciprocity between family members in either the kind or amount of care given or received. Indeed, the caregiving that takes place within the family unit underscores how meaningless it is to think in terms of a balanced distribution of resources among generations. At some points over the course of life we give more than we receive, but at other times the reverse is true. Moreover, we may receive far more from one relative than we will ever give to that individual, while the opposite may be true of our relationship with another relative. The exact extent or amount of the exchanges between any two family members is difficult, if not impossible, to measure, and an attempt at such measurement would be of dubious utility. Yet it is clear that these exchanges occur extensively and in great numbers and that they require considerable investments of personal resources.

FAMILY CAREGIVING
EVERYDAY AND EXTRAORDINARY

To understand the broad array of care provided by family members, it is useful to divide these exchanges into those that are "ordinary" and those that are "extraordinary" exchanges of care. The many ordinary, everyday transfers of care occur within families of every level of education or economic well-being, ethnic identity, race, or other identifying social or demographic characteristic. These are the exchanges that underlie the *interdependence* of the generations in the family, and, for the most part, family members want both to give and receive them. They come in a variety of forms: short-term and discrete, such as tending to a child's broken arm; of a few years' duration, such as diapering a baby or putting a young person through college; or of a considerable length of time, such as preparing breakfast for one's spouse day after day, for most of one's married life. Moreover, they may provide both maintenance support, for example, financial assistance, help with baby-sitting or shopping, and gift giving, or they may provide emotional support— expressions of, for example, affection, approval, or consolation (Kingson et al., 1986).

Family members also may find themselves called upon at some point to give or receive extraordinary care. This is assistance needed for an extended—indeed, often open-ended—period of time by individuals at *any* stage of the life course who have serious disabilities or illnesses. It is truly long-term care. Such care is required, for example, when a child is born with Down's Syndrome, when a spouse becomes a paraplegic as the result of an automobile accident, or when an elderly parent or grandparent develops a chronic and seriously debilitating heart ailment or suffers a severe stroke. Intergenerational exchanges of care under these circumstances also take place on a daily basis, but they usually are responses to more demanding support needs than ordinary caregiving tends to require. For instance, caregivers responding to extraordinary needs may find themselves helping the stricken family member to come to terms with chronic illness or disability, or with chronic pain, altered physical appearance, or limited capabilities. Often, continuous and comprehensive assistance with activities of daily living is required (Kingson et al., 1986).

It is primarily the family that responds when extraordinary support needs arise and, in most cases, bears the brunt of the ongoing costs. The opportunity to provide such support rarely is sought after by family members, for, certainly, when such support needs arise, they are likely to radically change the dynamics of both one's personal and family life—perhaps permanently. When faced with circumstances requiring extraordinary care, however, family members usually respond as well as they can for as long as they can (Kingson et al., 1986).

Providing long-term care for older family members with serious chronic illnesses or disabilities is one form of extraordinary caregiving affecting increasing numbers of American families. According to recent estimates (e.g., Manton, 1987, cited in Special Committee on Aging, 1987; Manton & Soldo, 1985) approximately 4 out of every 5 of the more than 6 million Americans who are 65 years of age or older and who require *some* level of

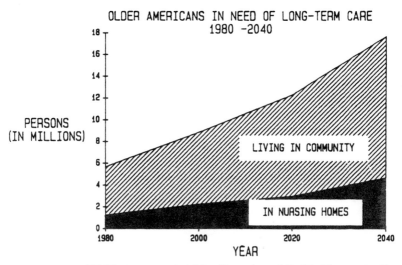

Figure 8.1. Older Americans in Need of Long-Term Care: 1980-2040

long-term care assistance live in a community setting rather than in a nursing home (see Figure 8.1). Moreover, data from the 1982 National Long-Term Care Survey indicate that about 19% of these community-based elderly are impeded from conducting normal activities because of their chronic conditions (Special Committee on Aging, 1987).

In the coming decades, even if the average age for the onset of disability conditions (such as severe arthritis and circulatory problems) was postponed several years, the number of elderly requiring long-term care is expected to increase. Current projections suggest that the *total* elderly long-term care population will increase to more than 9 million by the year 2000 and to nearly 19 million by 2040 (Manton & Soldo, 1985). If the current ratio of institutionalized to community-based chronic care elderly holds constant (approximately 1:4), that would mean *over 15 million* community-based chronic care elderly in 2040.

COSTS OF CAREGIVING TO FAMILY MEMBERS

The costs to family members resulting from responding to extraordinary care needs can be large, for this is "caregiving" with a big "C." Responsibilities related to the provision of such care often are stressful because they may not only test a family's caregiving abilities but also necessitate adjustments in all spheres of family life and in many aspects of individual behavior. In some cases the resulting stress can affect significantly the health and welfare of family members, particularly if substantial amounts of care are required of any one individual—usually the spouse or a daughter. These stresses fall into five general categories and are discussed below.

Demands on Time

Administering to a relative's care needs may take hours every day. In the process, it can reduce or eliminate the free time normally reserved for leisure activities or for personal needs. A study done in the 1970s by Newman and her colleagues at the Institute of Social Research at the University of Michigan found that two fifths of the children who provided parent care in their homes spent as much time caregiving as they would at a full-time job (Sandra Newman, James Morgan & Robert Marans, 1976). Data from the 1982 National Long-Term Care Survey/Survey of Caregivers found that, nationally, 31% of caregivers were employed while providing care. Almost 1 in 10 caregivers (9%) had to quit their jobs because of caregiving responsibilities (Stone, Cafferata, & Sangl, 1987). Research among three generations of women caregivers (Lang & Brody, 1983) showed that, as middle-aged women grow older, their caregiving responsibilities to parents increased. Women in their forties averaged 3 hours per week for caregiving tasks while those age 50 and older averaged more than 15 hours per week (Lang & Brody, 1983). This is consonant with the fact that many of the older women have older spouses whom they will care for and then survive, to live for some time in widowhood. Although the sample size was small and nonrandom, and thus possibly not representative nationally, these results are informative.

Demands on Space

In those cases where ill or disabled individuals and the caregiving family member(s) live together, the demands on physical space can be considerable. The care recipient often needs his or her own bedroom. Sometimes, special furniture or prosthetic devices may take up space in the living room, the kitchen, or the bathroom. Special foods and supplies may be in the refrigerator or in other storage areas common to all. However, even when the individual needing care does *not* live with caregiving family members, as in the example of a care-receiving parent who lives in the same community as a child does but not in the same residence, the latter may find their mobility limited and a compression of their daily geographical circuit. Moreover, travel plans are subject to the threat of curtailment or redesign, depending upon the ability of the chronically ill or disabled individual to handle change or temporary increases in self-sufficiency (Kingson et al., 1986). These issues often affect several members of a family indirectly as well—not just the primary caregiver.

Demands on Financial Resources

Caregiving can result in financial burdens. These are noted among marital dyads and also among caregivers who are parents or other family members. The marital bond also is an economic one, so the spouse is likely to feel great impact from the financial costs of long-term care. There are huge financial costs incurred when one spouse suffers a catastrophic illness, particularly when he or she must be institutionalized for an extended period of time (Kingson et al., 1986). Continuing chronic disease also can be very costly when medications, health care, and special devices or foods are considered. Families also may be affected by the need for a spouse caregiver who is in the workforce to take time off or reduce the number of hours on the job due to caregiving responsibilities. Indeed, when such responsibilities for a husband or a wife become so onerous that scheduling demands conflict frequently, they may impel working spouses to retire prior to when they would have otherwise and, thus, result in a considerable financial loss.

Financial costs can have serious intergenerational implications as well. For one thing, if the *personal* financial resources are reduced or eliminated, the subsequent financial support of a caregiver who survives his or (more probably) her spouse will likely become a family responsibility. In addition, older people who have considerably diminished or exhausted their personal resources in the process of taking care of their health needs are not likely to have financial assets to pass on to younger generations in the family (Kingson et al., 1986). Children often assume much of the financial burden of health services and care.

Psychological Stress

One of the greatest strains frequently facing family members providing long-term care is psychological stress. This can manifest itself in a variety of forms. One researcher has catalogued—among other manifestations— depression, anxiety, frustration, feelings of helplessness, sleeplessness, lowered morale, feelings of isolation, and feelings of conflict from having numerous responsibilities and from interference with life-style and social and recreational activities (Brody, 1981). The personification of adult children experiencing psychological stress, partially as a result of caregiving responsibilities for older parents, is the so-called "woman in the middle." She represents the women who

> are in middle age, in the middle from a generational standpoint, and in the middle in that the demands of their various roles compete for their time and energy. To an extent unprecedented in history, roles as paid workers and as care-giving daughters and daughters-in-law to dependent older people have been added to their traditional roles as wives, homemakers, mothers and grandmothers. (Brody, 1981, p. 471)

Physical Stress

It should come as no surprise that the "woman in the middle," as well as other individuals heavily involved in providing extraordinary care, may experience acute or chronic physical health problems themselves. Both the stress of competing demands and the process of providing the support itself require physical stamina. Moreover, often spouse caregivers, and even some of the child caregivers, may be feeling the effects of a diminished functional capacity themselves (Brody, 1981).

MOTIVATIONS FOR FAMILY CAREGIVING

Why do family members perform caregiving activities and aid ailing kin? Why do they continue to provide care, especially extraordinary care, frequently for an indefinite period? Possibly much of the persistence can be explained by factors that motivate close interpersonal relationships among family members. These factors individually or interactively impel the family to assume extraordinary responsibilities and "stay with it." They are intrinsic to either the family as a whole or to the dynamic between one particular family caregiver and one particular care recipient. Included in this category are psychological bonding, intergenerational family solidarity, societal norms, reciprocity, and continuity of generations.

Psychological Bonding

The most fundamental of psychological attachments involves the bonding of family members to each other. Bonds of husbands to wife, parent to child, and sibling to sibling based upon feelings of love, affection, intimacy, and nurturance, as well as upon both the positive and negative facets of relation-ships that involve dependency on others, are common to all. Also, an important component of ego development is the ability to see oneself as reflected in those with whom one is involved in an intimate relationship. Providing care for a loved one who must contend with the difficulties of adjusting to diminished autonomy and then observing the outcome of this process (successful or otherwise) can lead to a greater insight into oneself (Cantor & Hirshorn, 1986).

Intergenerational Family Solidarity

Closely connected to the psychological bonding that occurs within the context of the family are the various kinds of familial solidarity, particularly between generations, that the family as a social unit usually engenders. Families display intergenerational solidarity in a number of ways. Among them is *associational* solidarity, which refers to the extent and nature of the interactions between family members, for example, recreation, conversation, family rituals, and gatherings (see Bengtson & Burton, 1980, 1973, 1980; Bengtson & Schrader, 1982; Sussman, 1965, 1976, 1977; Troll, 1971; Troll, Miller, & Atchely, 1979). There also is *affectual* solidarity, which refers to the amount and nature of the positive sentiment (e.g., warmth, closeness, emotional gratification) present in the family (see Bengtson & Black, 1973; Cantor, 1976). Also considered an aspect of solidarity between the genera-tions in the family is *consensus*—or the amount of agreement or disagree-ment--regarding value systems, beliefs, and perspectives (see Bengtson, 1970, 1975; Hill, Foote, Aldous, Carlson, & MacDonald, 1970). A high degree of consensus within a family indicates common, intrafamilial norms that frequently exist despite the fact that family members of different gener-ations have widely divergent levels of education, life-styles, or political orientations (Cantor & Hirshorn, 1986).

Societal Norms

Norms held widely on a societal level interact with the dynamics of family life to affect intergenerational caregiving. These norms comprise the moral, ethical, and religious directives that regulate relations between the genera-tions in most families. They include unwritten or written rules regarding filial responsibility such as the Biblical dictum to "Honor thy father and thy mother" or laws regulating bequests upon the death of parents. Most cultures have unwritten laws in this domain that serve as particularly strong incen-tives. For example, while filial responsibility, "the responsibility of children to care for their aged parents before or instead of the government or charitable institutions," (Schorr, 1980) is no longer a legal obligation in the United States; it is an internalized, motivating force for many children of frail parents in this country. The importance of different societal norms as motivators of family caregiving varies considerably from culture to culture and, particularly, among ethnic groups. (Illustrative examples can be found in Fandetti & Gelfand, 1976; Gelfand & Kutzik, 1979; Guemple, 1983; Johnson, 1977, 1979, 1983; Plath, 1973).

Reciprocity in Exchanges Between Family Members

Reciprocity between family members is based on a complex series of interactions that have occurred over an extended period of time and that depend heavily on perceptions of how much the individuals involved gave or received in the past. The concept of reciprocity as a process that occurs at various points along the life course reinforces the idea that most frail elderly individuals who are the recipients of care from family members both have given resources to and received resources from family members for quite some time. Researchers have woven the lifecourse framework for family exchanges into theories that variously perceive reciprocity in terms of relative amounts of power in a relationship (Blau, 1964; Dowd, 1975; Weber, 1947); fairness in the distribution of family property (e.g., Bengtson & Treas, 1980; Cates & Sussman, 1982; Sussman, Cates, & Smith, 1970); or, in the case of older people specifically, in terms of "credits earned" for providing assistance in the past to those now serving as their caregivers (Horowitz & Shindleman, 1983).

Continuity/Discontinuity of the Generations

For many families, the caregiving and receiving process is infused with mores and values that have been passed down through the generations. Thus, for example, in some families the care-*giving* activities an adult child performs for a frail parent provide, as well, a template for the care-*receiving* that that child expects in frail old age from his or her own children. (Kingson et al., 1986; Cantor & Hirshorn, 1986).

Not all caregivers, however, come away from the experience of providing care for a spouse or parent with the desire to see their own experience repeated by their children. In a nonrepresentative sample of 403 Philadelphia-area women concerning opinions regarding what adult children should do to help a dependent parent, Brody and her associates found that there was some variation, along generational lines, in personal preferences for service providers in their own old age. For instance, while about one half of the women who were in the "grandmother" generation would prefer to have their children help with expenses if they were to experience frailty in old age, only 14% of the "middle generation" women would want their children to perform this task, preferring formal support from pensions or insurance instead. Similar patterns emerged for other types of caregiving activities (Brody, Johnsen, & Fulcomer, 1984). There is abundant anecdotal evidence, as well, from medical and social service clinicians, that some adult children find certain aspects of their caregiving experience sufficiently negative that they are determined to interact differently with their own children should they themselves face a frail old age (e.g., make a different set of demands; try to rely more heavily on formal sources of support). In such cases, the caregiving/care-receiving experience serves as a catalyst for change as well as a focal point for familial interaction.

In considering caregiving in families within the intergenerational transfer model, several points were made. It is important to note that ordinary and extraordinary caregiving and receiving occur across the life course in a family context. Despite costs of care provision to the family member, the process continues. Much of the motivation may derive from intergenerational aspects of family life.

Analyzing caregiving as such can be very helpful, especially with regard to extraordinary caregiving. This can serve as an indicator of much that is positive or negative about the family as a social entity as well as about any one family in particular. Worth watching in the coming years, given the growing proportion of the total population in the seventh decade of life and older, will be the response of a concomitantly increasing number of families facing the care needs of their older family members. In particular, the following questions come to mind: How will families handle the attendant costs described above? Will they demand greater public sector support? Will changes in family structure, including those resulting from a substantial decrease in the birth rate, *force* a greater public sector response? Undoubtedly, Americans will have to confront these issues, on both the societal and the personal level, as we move into the 21st century.

REFERENCES

Bengtson, V. L. (1970). The generation gap: A review and typology of social-psychological perspectives. *Youth and Society, 2,* 7-21.

Bengtson, V. L. (1975). Generation and family effects in value socialization. *American Sociological Review, 40,* 358-371.

Bengtson, V. L., & Black, K. D. (1973). Intergenerational relations and continuities in social-ization. In P. Baltes & W. Schaie (Eds.), *Life-span developmental psychology: Personality and socialization.* New York: Van Nostrand Reinhold.

Bengtson, V. L., & Burton, L. (1980, November). *Families and support systems among three ethnic groups.* Paper presented at the 33rd annual meeting of the Gerontological Society of America, San Diego, CA.

Bengtson, V. L., & Schrader, S. (1982). Parent-child relations. In D. J. Mangen & W. A. Peterson (Eds.), *Research instruments in social gerontology* (Vol. 2). Minneapolis: University of Minnesota Press.

Bengtson, V. L., & Treas, J. (1980). The changing family context of mental health and aging. In J. E. Birren & R. B. Sloane (Eds.), *Handbook of mental health and aging.* Englewood Cliffs, NJ: Prentice-Hall.

Blau, P. M. (1964). *Exchanges and power in social life.* New York: John Wiley.

Brody, E. M. (1981). Parent care as a normative family stress. *The Gerontologist, 21*(5), 477.

Brody, E. M., Johnsen, P. T., & Fulcomer, M. C. (1984). What should adult children do for elderly parents? Opinions and preferences of three generations of women. *Journal of Gerontology, 39*(5), 736-746.

Cantor, M. H. (1976). *The configuration and intensity of the informal support system in a New York City elderly population.* Paper presented at the annual meeting of the Gerontological Society of America, New York.

Cantor, M. H., & Hirshorn, B. A. (1986, November). *Intergenerational transfers within the family context--Motivating factors and their implications for caregiving.* Paper presented at the annual meeting of the Gerontological Society of America, Chicago.

Cates, J. N., & Sussman, M. B. (1982). Family systems and inheritance. In J. N. Cates & M. B. Sussman (Eds.), *Family systems and inheritance patterns* (pp. 1-24). New York: Haworth.

Dowd, J. J. (1975). Aging as exchange: A preface to theory. *Journal of Gerontology, 30*(5), 584-594.

Fandetti, D. V., & Gelfand, D. E. (1976). Care of the aged: Attitudes of white ethnic families. *The Gerontologist, 16,* 544-549.

Gelfand, D. E., & A. J. Kutzik (Eds.). (1979). *Ethnicity and aging.* New York: Springer.

Guemple, L. (1983). Growing old in Inuit society. In J. Sokolovsky (Ed.), *Growing old in different societies: Cross-cultural perspectives* (pp. 24-28). Belmont, CA: Wadsworth.

Hill, R., Foote, N., Aldous, J., Carlson, R., & MacDonald, R. (1970). *Family development in three generations.* Cambridge, MA: Schenkman.

Horowitz, A., & Shindleman, L. W. (1983). Reciprocity and affection: Past influences on current caregiving. *Journal of Gerontological Social Work, 5*(3), 6.

Johnson, C. L. (1977). Interdependence, reciprocity and indebtedness: An analysis of Japanese American kinship relations. *Journal of Marriage and the Family, 39*(5), 351-362.

Johnson, C. L. (1979). Family support systems to elderly Italian Americans. *Journal of Minority Aging, 3*(1), 34-41.

Johnson, C. L. (1983). Interdependence and aging in Italian families. In J. Sokolovsky (Ed.), *Growing old in different societies: Cross-cultural perspectives* (pp. 92-103). Belmont, CA: Wadsworth.

Kane, R. L., & Kane, R. A. (1981). *Assessing the elderly* (p. 19). Lexington, MA: Lexington.

Kaufman, A. (1980, March). Social policy and long-term care of the aged. *Social Work,* 134-137.

Kingson, E. R., Hirshorn, B. A., & Cornman, J. M. (1986). *Ties that bind, The interdependence of generations.* Cabin John, MD: Seven Locks.

Lang, A. M., & Brody, E. M. (1983). Characteristics of middle-aged daughters and help to their elderly mothers. *Journal of Marriage and the Family,* 197.

Liu, K., & Manton, K. (1987). Long-term care: Current estimates and projections, 1987. *Developments in aging: 1987, Vol. 3* (Report 100-291). Washington, DC: Government Printing Office.

Manton, K. G., & Soldo, B. J. (1985). Dynamics of health changes in the oldest old. *Milbank Memorial Fund Quarterly/Health and Society, 63*,(2).

Newman, S., Morgan, J., & Marans, R. (1976). *Housing adjustments of older people: A report of findings from the second phase.* Ann Arbor: University of Michigan, Institute for Social Research.

Plath, D. W. (1973). Ecstasy years—Old age in Japan. *Pacific Affairs, 46,* 421-428.

Ripley, R. B., & Franklin, F. A. (1979). *Congress, the bureaucracy and public policy* (2nd ed.). Homewood, IL: Dorsey.

Schorr, A. (1980). *Honor thy father and thy mother: A second look at filial responsibility and family policy.* Washington, DC: Social Security Administration.

Shanas, E. (1973). Family-kin networks and aging in cross-cultural perspective. *Journal of Marriage and the Family, 35,* 505-511.

Shanas, E. (1980). Older people and their families: The new pioneers. *Journal of Marriage and the Family, 42*(1), 9-15.

Special Committee on Aging-United States Senate. (1986). *Developments in aging: 1986, Vol. 1* (S. Doc. 100-8). Washington, DC: Government Printing Office.

Special Committee on Aging-United States Senate. (1987). *Developments in aging: 1987, Vol. 1* (Report No. 100-291). Washington, DC: Government Printing Office.

Stone, R., Cafferata, G. L., & Sangl, J. (1987). Caregivers of the frail elderly: A national profile. *The Gerontologist, 27*(5), 622.

Sussman, M. B. (1965). Relationships of adult children with their parents in the United States. In E. Shanas & G. Streib (Eds.), *Social structure and the family: Generational relations.* Englewood Cliffs, NJ: Prentice-Hall.

Sussman, M. B. (1976). The family life of old people. In R. H. Binstock & E. Shanas (Eds.), *Handbook of aging and the social sciences* (pp. 218-243). New York: Van Nostrand Reinhold.

Sussman, M. B. (1977). *Incentives and family environments for the elderly.* Washington, DC: Administration on Aging.

Sussman, M. B., Cates, J., & Smith, D. (1970). *The family of inheritance.* New York: Russell Sage.

Troll, L. E. (1971). The family of later life: A decade review. *Journal of Marriage and the Family, 33,* 263-290.

Troll, L. E., Miller, S., & Atchley, R. (1979). *Families in later life.* Belmont, CA: Wadsworth.

Weber, M. (1947). *The theory of social and economic organization.* New York: Oxford University Press.

Chapter 9

FAMILY IMPLICATIONS OF HEART DISEASE AMONG THE ELDERLY

ROSALIE F. YOUNG

There are immense family implications of heart disease, particularly among the elderly. At later life, heart conditions are prevalent; furthermore, they serve as major sources of disability. More than 20% of older persons have suffered heart attacks. One fourth the activity limitation of older persons is due to heart disease, and this chronic condition is responsible for the largest amount of hospital days, physician visits, and bed disability days of persons over the age of 65 (U.S. Department of Health and Human Services, 1986).

On the personal and familial level, heart disease poses a major threat to the life quality and well-being of patients and their families (Krantz & Deckel, 1983). The experience of a major heart problem such as myocardial infarction (MI) has two important family implications. First, since this sudden, life-threatening cardiac event has consequences for the mortality, morbidity, and functioning consequences of the older patient, it directly threatens the security and emotional state of his or her family. Second, because much of the care and out-of-hospital management of this most

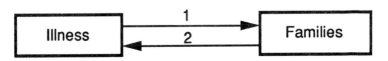

Figure 9.1. The Family-Illness Intermesh

serious illness occurs in the family setting, a caregiving situation begins that can involve considerable family commitment.

This basic premise reflects the focus of the chapter—that there is an intermesh of families and illness that is mutual. This family-illness intermesh is illustrated in Figure 9.1.

The family-illness intermesh is conceptualized as the mutual impact of illness on the family unit and of families upon the illness situation. As shown by Arrow 1 in Figure 9.1, illness is extraindividual in its effect; it affects family members as well as patients. The reverse process, illustrated in Figure 9.1 by Arrow 2, indicates that the family can exert influence over the illness situation and the recovery process. Using their resources, families can have considerable influence over the health/illness continuum. Application of this model affords explanation of how illness may strain families and how the family can be considered a proactive, rather than reactive unit, when faced with disease (Young, 1985).

Implied by the family-illness intermesh model is that the family caregiver plays an essential role in illness situations. He or she is directly affected by the health problem but can have considerable influence on the outcomes. Thus the model can be elaborated to include the role of the caregiver, as shown in Figure 9.2.

In considering the impact of MI, the illness-outcomes model can be helpful. The general aftermath of this sudden, life-threatening condition includes poor physical functioning, considerable fatigue, and major emotional stress to the patient. These effects often are intensified among the elderly (Bergner, Bergner, Hallstrom, Eisenberg, & Cobb, 1984; Croog & Levine, 1982). The physical reserve of older persons is reduced, and they are less able to have sustained bodily response to a major illness stressor (Finlayson & McEwen, 1977; Hickey, 1980). For the patient and family (Arrows 1 and 2 of Figure 9.2), there is the period of immediate crisis. During this acute phase the concerns of all are on survival. Following this initial period, there is the time of adjustment to hospitalization and observation of the patient's progress. Often during the course of hospitalization, there is a bout of depression on the part of patients as they come to grips with their mortality; fears of disability surface. After patients are discharged from the

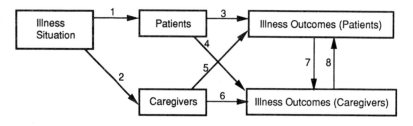

Figure 9.2. Patient, Family, and Illness Outcomes

hospital, personal and familial effects may be exacerbated. In the immediate post hospital stage, patient fatigue and mood swings on the one hand, and caregiver services and caregiver anxiety on the other, create a difficult situation for all. Patients may become depressed or anxious (diGiacomo, 1981; Gruen, 1975; Hackett & Cassem, 1975; Wishnie, Hackett, & Cassem, 1971). The mental health aftereffects of a major heart problem can be as damaging as the heart condition itself. Fears of recurrence, anxiety about survival, worries about job, sexual functioning, and dependency are all common. Some heart patients exhibit great fear about resuming activities and become cardiac invalids (Badura & Waltz, 1984). While capable of functioning in many areas, their fears are sufficient to keep them bedridden. At later stages, anxious and/or depressed patients often die.

As the recovering patient experiences physical and mental distress, the family worries about his or her symptoms, how complete their recovery will be, and shares the patient's fears of dependency. Often, while they aid the patient and help facilitate life-style changes that may be required, caregivers also become depressed or anxious. In general, the early home phase of recovery is an adjustment phase; both the patient and the family must adapt to the patient's impaired physical functioning, dependency, and possible mental health aftereffects, as well as to life-style and behavioral changes required by the heart attack.

As an adjustment phase, positive responses often emerge. Individual and family resources are marshalled, and coping strategies emerge (Doherty & Campbell, 1988). As illustrated in Figure 9.2 by Arrows 3 and 4, both patients and their family caregivers play crucial roles in facilitating patient recuperation. Indeed, the family caregiver is most salient to restoration of the heart patient's health and mental well-being, and to preventing recurrence of heart problems. Unfortunately, this role often is linked to adverse caregiver effects (Croog & Fitzgerald, 1978; Croog & Levine, 1982). Physical or mental health may suffer, and the caregiver's social activity and personal time declines dramatically. Indeed, two thirds of heart patient wives have been observed to have adverse mental health effects (Croog & Levine, 1982). Thus the physical process of aiding, and the psychological strain of watching a loved one endure a major heart problem converge, and the caregiver may suffer. Difficult patients may provide more strain to the caregiver. The caregiver also may contribute to the stress he or she is under by poor coping, negative attitudes, or other counterproductive personal behaviors (see Figure 9.2, Arrows 5 and 6).

Consistent with the contention that there are many adverse caregiver effects is an expectation that is not always stated, but often assumed. Patient progress seems to imply negative caregiver effects. Visualizing this in terms of the illness outcomes model, it is believed that (a) patient-caregiver outcomes are related (see Figure 9.2, Arrows 7 and 8), and (b) that strain, burden, or burnout among caregivers is the result of care but related to patient recuperation. Consequences to the caregiver are the price paid for patient recovery or stability. An asymmetrical outcome situation is posed. This patient recovery/caregiver strain model influences our thinking and often is corroborated by research findings.

Actually, this scenario is only one of four possible outcomes. Because the patient and caregiver are ensconced in a mutual situation, and outcomes particular to one affect the outcomes of the other, there are four likely outcomes as follows: (1) patient prospers while caregiver declines; (2) caregiver thrives but patient declines; (3) both members of the dyad prosper; (4) both decline. Thus there is the possibility of symmetrical *or* asymmetrical outcomes; furthermore, these may be positive *or* negative. The four outcomes are depicted in Figure 9.3 in terms of typology.

All four outcomes have been noted in the literature. Most research, however, supports the patterns denoted in cells B, C, and D, that there are adverse effects to one or both. In recognition of the strain to caregivers, there are programmatic efforts to provide them with respite care as they aid patients in recuperation or help to stabilize the patient's condition (cell C); see, for example, Gallagher, Lovett, and Zeiss, (1989); Lawton and Brody, (1984); Montgomery, (1989); and Paradis, (1988). Coppel, Burton, Becker, and Fiore (1985); Poulshock and Deimling (1984), and Zarit, Todd, and Zarit (1986) have associated poor mental and physical health states among patients and corresponding adverse caregiver mental health states (cell D). Sometimes the patient suffers mental or physical abuse at the hands of the caregiver (cell B); see, for example, Bernatavicz, (1982), and Wolf, (1984).

Although the literature is sparsest regarding a positive trajectory among patients and caregivers, there is some evidence of dyadic progress (cell A).

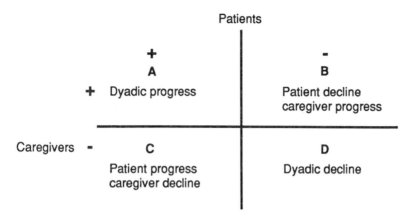

Figure 9.3. Typology of Patient-Caregiver Illness Outcomes

Patients recover, caregivers are emotionally relieved and relinquish the caregiving role, and both are observed to be adjusting well. Indeed, half of the heart patient-caregiver dyads interviewed in a study of 183 family units were found to have mental health symptomatology scores in the normal range (Young & Kahana, 1987). Both patients and their caregivers were shown to be functioning well one year after a late-life heart attack. Furthermore, studies have shown many examples of caregivers whose caregiving experiences can be characterized as "beneficial" rather than "burdensome." The process of caring for a loved one can be rewarding and can contribute to a mutually satisfying relationship between patient and care provider (Sangl, 1985). For many, there is gratification from the service role and the belief that the care provision efforts are helpful to the patient's recovery (Kinney & Stephens, 1989; Masciocchi, Thomas, & Moeller, 1984).

Proposing that divergent outcomes may result from the same type of major health problem suggests that there are specific factors that can contribute to any or all of the end points. Within the context of the overall conceptualization of the caregiving paradigm, the four dyadic outcomes denoted in the typology can be considered as part of a dynamic model (Young & Kahana, 1987). According to this model, the several factors that determine good versus bad outcomes for one or both members of the dyad include (a) circumstances particular to each of the individuals, to the illness, and to the caregiving situation; (b) the resources of each dyadic member; and (c) the interaction between dyadic units (see Figure 9.4).

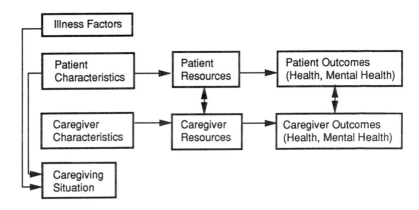

Figure 9.4. Caregiving Outcomes Model

Thus, according to the caregiving outcomes model, recovery for the patient and also well-being for the caregiver (positive family effects) are conceptualized as the result of several major elements. Specific variables that comprise the elements can include the following:

(1) Patient sociodemographic characteristics
(2) Patient attitudinal, personality, and illness behavior variables, including attitude toward caregiver and caregiving
(3) Caregiver sociodemographic characteristics
(4) Caregiver attitudinal and personality variables, including interpretation of patient recovery and dependency role
(5) Illness characteristics, including symptoms and treatment needs
(6) Caregiving situation characteristics including environmental context of site, whether single or joint caregiver, and amount and length of caregiving
(7) Patient resources, including coping strategies, social support, and economic variables
(8) Caregiver resources, including coping strategies, social support, and economic variables
(9) Patient-caregiver interaction variables, including cohesive and empathic interactions

When considering the family impact of serious late-life illness, the model proposed may be quite useful. As shown, it is based upon the premise that there is an important interface between families and illness situations. In addition, the family-illness intermesh can be mutual in that families can affect the outcomes and be crucial to producing good aftereffects. Further, caregiving outcomes for patients and their family care providers relate to each other; neither exists independently of the other. Finally, there are important factors that can determine whether the family as a unit or the individual members of the patient-caregiver dyad fare well after a serious health problem such as MI.

There are important applications of this model for human and health service providers. One possible application might be to assist health providers in predicting which patients might fare well after hospital discharge, insofar as receiving family care is concerned. If variables such as those included in the model are used in constructing a screening tool, each patient can be assessed for level of recovery-enhancing resources. It is then possible to determine whether patients have a caregiver who will provide aid; if they have additional sources of social support; whether they are of a personality type that is likely to respond negatively to disability, interact favorably with their care providers, and so forth. Similarly, the caregiver's ability to withstand the strains of care is affected by whether his or her attitudes or preexisting health problems are likely to make caregiving difficult (i.e., whether he or she is an at-risk aid provider). These determinations could be quite helpful to discharge planners because they could facilitate better outcomes among both patients and family caregivers.

Those of us involved in the field of gerontology are keenly aware of the need to have better tools to serve the ailing aged. These pertain to medical techniques, to a more extensive range of services and, also, to the ability of the informal sector to aid and assist during or after a major health problem. If we consider the aftermath of a major health problem within the context of an overall approach to the family-illness intermesh and then try to determine the best circumstances for care, we than can better understand and better aid older patients and their families. It is most essential that we realize the factors that contribute to poor outcomes of elderly illness for both the patient and the family and then investigate how to shore up the family caregiver. This will enable both the patient and the care provider to endure this difficult experience without undue stress.

REFERENCES

Badura, B., & Waltz, M. (1984). Social support and the quality of life following myocardial infarction. *Social Indicators Research, 14,* 295-311.

Bergner, L., Bergner, M., Hallstrom, A. P., Eisenberg, M., & Cobb, L. A. (1984). Health status of survivors of out-of-hospital cardiac arrest six months later. *American Journal of Public Health, 74,* 508-510.

Bernatavicz, F. (1982). Family, neighbors and friends. *Improving protective services for older Americans*. Portland: Human Services Development Institute, University of Southern Maine.

Coppel, D. B., Burton, C., Becker, J., & Fiore, J. (1985). Relationships of cognitions associated with coping reactions to depression in spousal caregivers of Alzheimer's disease patients. *Cognitive Therapy and Research, 9,* 253-266.

Croog, S., & Fitzgerald, E. (1978). Subjective stress and serious illness of a spouse: Wives of heart patients. *Journal of Health and Social Behavior, 19,* 166-178.

Croog, S., & Levine, S. (1982). *Life after a heart attack: Social and psychological factors eight years later.* New York: Human Sciences Press.

diGiacomo, J. N. (1981). Psychiatric aspects of the cardiac patient. *Mount Sinai Journal of Medicine, 48,* 543-551.

Doherty, W. J., & Campbell, T. L. (1988). *Families and health.* Newbury Park, CA: Sage.

Finlayson, A., & McEwen, J. (1977). *Coronary heart disease and patterns of living.* New York: Prodist.

Gallagher, D., Lovett, S., & Zeiss, A. (1989). Interventions with caregivers of frail elderly persons. In M. Ory & K. Bond (Eds.), *Aging and health care* (pp. 167-190). New York: Routledge.

Gruen, W. (1975). Effects of brief psychotherapy during the hospitalization period on the recovery process in heart attacks. *Journal of Consulting and Clinical Psychology, 43,* 232-233.

Hackett, T. P., & Cassem, N. H. (1975). Psychological management of the myocardial infarction patient. *Journal of Human Stress, 1,* 25-38.

Hickey, T. (1980). *Health and aging.* Monterey, CA: Brooks/Cole.

Kinney, J. M., & Stephens, M.A.P. (1989). Hassles and uplifts of giving care to a family member with dementia. *Psychology and Aging, 4,* 402-408.

Krantz, D. S., & Deckel, A. W. (1983). *Coping with chronic disease: Research and applications.* New York: Academic Press.

Lawton, M. P., & Brody, E. M. (1984). *A multiservice respite program for family caregivers of patients with Alzheimer's disease.* Research program funded by the Pew Foundation and the Hartford Foundation to the Philadelphia Geriatric Center, Philadelphia, PA.

Masciocchi, C., Thomas, A., & Moeller, T. (1984). Support for the impaired elderly: A challenge for family care-givers. In Q. William & G. A. Hughston (Eds.), *Independent aging: Family and social systems* (pp. 115-131). Rockville, MD: Aspen Systems.

Montgomery, R. J. V. (1989). Investigating caregiver burden. In K. S. Markides & C. L. Cooper (Eds.), *Aging, stress and health.* New York: John Wiley.

Paradis, L. F. (1988). *Stress and burnout among providers caring for the terminally ill and their families.* New York: Haworth.

Poulshock, S. W. & Deimling, G. T. (1984). Families caring for elders in residences: Issues in the measurement of burden. *Journal of Gerontology, 39,* 230-239.

Sangl, J. (1985). The family support system of the elderly. In R. Vogel & H. Palmer (Eds.), *Long term care: Perspectives from research and demonstration* (pp. 307-336). Rockville, MD: Aspen Systems.

U.S. Department of Health and Human Services. (1986). Current estimates from the National Health Interview Survey, United States, 1984. *Vital and health statistics* (Series 10, No. 156, DHHS Publication No. PHS 86-1584). Washington, DC: Government Printing Office.

Wishnie, H. A., Hackett, T. P., & Cassem, N. H. (1971). Psychological hazards of convalescence following myocardial infarction. *Journal of the American Medical Association, 215,* 1292-1296.

Wolf, R. S. (1984). *Elder abuse and neglect: Final report from three model projects.* Worcester: University of Massachusetts Medical Center, University Center on Aging.

Young, R. F. (1985). *Mental health, adaptation and care of aged* (USPHS Grant No. 1R01-AG05248). Washington, DC: National Institute of Health.

Young, R., & Kahana, E. (1987). Conceptualizing stress, coping, and illness management in heart disease caregiving. *The Hospice Journal, 3,* 53-73.

Zarit, S., Todd, P., & Zarit, J. (1986). Subjective burden of husbands and wives as caregivers: A longitudinal study. *The Gerontologist, 26,* 260-266.

Chapter 10

UNDERSTANDING CAREGIVING INTERVENTIONS IN THE CONTEXT OF THE STRESS MODEL

EVA KAHANA
JENNIFER KINNEY

After two decades of research on the stresses of caring for a dependent older adult, research in this area is at a crossroads. On one hand, those of us who conduct research in the area of caregiving stress have come a long way. We now know with a fair degree of certainty approximately how many people are caring for an older family member; demographically we can "describe" the typical caregiver, and we can discuss in great detail the challenges these caregivers face as they balance their caregiving role with other roles such as wife, mother, and professional (Biegel & Blum, 1988-1989). We also have documented a litany of caregivers' reactions to their caregiving responsibilities, including feelings of burden and both psychiatric (e.g., depression, anxiety, hostility, affect) and physical (e.g., health service utilization, sick days, nutritional and immuninological assays, sleep problems) symptoms. (For recent reviews, see Schulz, 1990; Toseland & Smith, in press.) On the other hand, we are not yet in a position to share with caregiving families a formula that will help eliminate the negative aspects and consequences of their caregiving roles. For practitioners and policy-makers, this poses a major challenge as they seek systematic guidelines for assisting caregivers of the growing number of frail elderly.

In part, our dilemma reflects our ambitiousness. Caregiving stress research, by its very nature, constantly reminds us of the interplay between theory and practice. Some of us began studying caregiving with the intent of contributing to theories of chronic stress. Others among us became involved in caregiving research because we saw, through our practices, the devastation that caregiving can cause. Through our involvement, we have found that we very much need each other. Development of theories of caregiving stress requires an understanding of the "human" side of caregiving; similarly, we need theories of stress before we can design interventions to promote greater well-being among family caregivers. In this chapter, we conceptualize caregiving within the larger stress-theoretic framework and discuss implications of this conceptualization for intervention strategies. We propose a conceptual model of the impact of caregiving stress that may help organize caregiving intervention in terms of the components of the stress model that they affect.

WHAT CAN INTERVENTIONS OFFER?

Researchers in the area of caregiving stress have amply documented the stressful nature of caregiving (e.g., Anthony-Bergstone, Zarit, & Gaitz, 1988; Brody, 1981; Poulshock & Deimling, 1984; Zarit, Orr, & Zarit, 1985), despite claims by some researchers that caregiving arrangements can benefit both patient and caregiver (e.g., Danis, 1978; Johnson, 1988; Moss, Lawton, Dean, Goodman, & Schneider, 1987; Seelbach, 1978). Recently, several caregiving researchers have suggested that, having documented the existence of both positive and negative caregiving situations, it is time to turn our attention to identifying those less-than-optimal caregiving situations for which interventions might exist and to offer these interventions in a timely fashion so that they are of maximum benefit (Teri, 1990; Zarit, 1990). We believe that prior to intervening in a caregiving situation, professionals must consider (a) whether intervention is necessary; (b) what aspect of the caregiving situation should be modified; (c) what type of intervention is most likely to be effective; (d) who should intervene; (e) when is the appropriate time for intervention; and (f) what are the likely consequences of intervention. In an effort to clarify the complexity of caregiving, and the inherent difficulty of intervening in this process, first we will place caregiving stress in a larger theoretical perspective and then present a model of stress that will help to organize our discussion of caregiving interventions, their impact, and potential effectiveness.

THE STRESS PARADIGM

Current conceptualizations of caregiving stress adopt a transactional or process approach (e.g., Kahana & Kahana, 1984; Lazarus & Folkman, 1984; Pearlin, 1983; Pearlin, Turner, & Semple, 1989). These models of stress maintain that stress is a process. That is, stress is not static but rather evolves and unfolds over time. Lazarus and Folkman conceptualize the stress process as an ongoing series of interactions among objective events in the environment, individuals' appraisals (perceptions) of these events, attempts to cope with these appraisals, and behavioral and psychosocial outcomes. Pearlin and colleagues conceptualize the stress process as comprising three domains: stressors (objective and subjective), mediators (including coping and social support), and outcomes. Stress also can be thought of as a "mismatch" between a person and his or her environment (Kahana & Kahana, 1984). Regardless of the specific perspective, each of these theorists believes that the components of each stress model are dynamically related and that change in one part of the model will result in changes in the other parts of the model. In addition to recognizing complexities involved in transactions that define stress and its impact on caregivers, recent conceptualizations have also acknowledged the importance of considering roles of both caregiver and care recipient characteristics, and of dyadic relationships between caregivers and care recipients, as influencing caregiver outcomes (Kahana & Young, 1990; Young & Kahana, 1987). Given the interrelatedness of these transactional models, and the complexity they afford, they offer a good framework for the consideration of the complexity of caregiving interventions.

A caregiving model that incorporates dynamic elements of the general stress models and extends them to the specific dimensions of stress and resources most salient to caregiving intervention is presented in Figure 10.1

This model acknowledges some of the complexities of the caregiving paradigm that have been suggested both by recent empirical studies and conceptualizations of the stress paradigm. In this model, the stress process consists of three major components: (a) sources of stress, (b) resources, and (c) outcomes. Accordingly, it incorporates the major notions from the three models of stress presented above. Our model acknowledges the importance of appraisals of stress along with objective components of stress associated

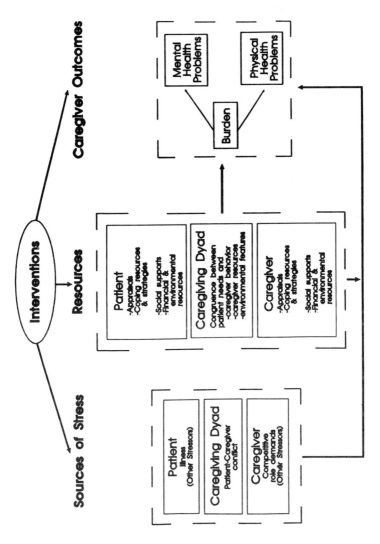

Figure 10.1. Conceptual Model of Interventions Relevant to Caregiving Stress

with caregiving; it incorporates noncaregiving demands and responsibilities faced by caregivers, and it allows for resources to intervene between stress and caregivers' well-being. In specifying sources of stress and resources, we consider those attributable to caregiver characteristics, those attributable to care recipient characteristics, and those based on the relationship between caregivers and care recipients.

The model identifies three major sources of stress. The first source of stress arises from the care recipient's illness/disability (e.g., degree of impairment, behavior problems, and the amount of assistance required in basic and instrumental activities of daily living). In Pearlin's model, these stressors can be thought of as objective, primary stressors. Pearlin also posits secondary stressors that are based on the caregivers interpretations or appraisals of primary stressors. Our model presents a noteworthy departure from Pearlin's conceptualizations of stress. In our model we include appraisals under coping resources rather than considering them as stressors. We believe that it is most useful to classify appraisals of the patient's illness as representing coping with the objective stress. Negative appraisals may constitute a secondary stress whereas positive appraisals may represent a resource. In terms of interventions, we find it useful to distinguish between objective sources of stress that largely are external to actions and responses of the caregiver, and behavioral or intrapsychic responses to those stressors that we consider to be personal coping resources or strategies.

The second set of major stressors in our model refers to objective demands made on the caregiver that may pose problems due to his or her caregiving roles. They relate to aspects of a caregiver's life that become affected by caregiving over time, such as responsibilities to children, job and financial worries, or social life restriction. Finally, we consider aspects of the caregiver's dyadic interactions with the care recipient that present problems or contribute to interpersonal conflict between caregiver and care recipient as comprising a major source of stress.

Caregiving stress models propose that the influence of stressors on caregivers' mental and physical health is buffered by resources. In our model, possible resources include personal, social, and environmental resources available not only to the caregiver but also to the person for whom he or she is caring. Personal resources might include coping strategies used by both a caregiver and the care recipient and the ways in which they appraise their situation(s). Social resources include friends and family members who assist the caregiver, care recipient, or both; environmental resources include, among others, finances and the living environment of the caregiving dyad. Our model proposes that the resources available to a caregiving dyad can help to offset the negative consequences to caregivers' health and well-being that sometimes result from caregiving stresses. Kahana and Kahana (1984) suggest that, to the extent that there is a "fit" or "match" between the demands presented by the stress and the available resources, caregivers' well-being will not be negatively affected. For example, to the extent that the caregiver provides appropriate levels of assistance to the care recipient with activities of daily living (neither too little nor too much), the caregiver's well-being will be harmonized.

The final component of our model consists of caregiving outcomes. To the extent that there is a mismatch between stresses and resources, caregivers will feel burdened, and mental and physical distress will result. We conceptualize burden as caregivers' feelings that they are overwhelmed with caregiving and include burden as an outcome in our model to reinforce our belief that caregivers' perceptions of and evaluations of their situation determine which caregivers will experience difficulty in their role as a caregiver. Our model also considers objectively observable health or mental problems among caregivers as ultimate consequences of caregiver burden.

We believe that this model serves as a useful heuristic for conceptualizing caregiving interventions in terms of (a) where in the stress process they occur, (b) the component of the stress process they attempt to modify, and (c) the impact they have on other aspects of the process. There are several additional advantages of such a model. First, by distinguishing objective from subjective stressors—that is, by acknowledging the role of appraisal in the stress process—we are reminded of the importance of individual difference among the caregivers we serve. We cannot assume that all caregivers have the same needs or that they feel the same way about the things they do for the care recipient. In fact, what serves as a stressor for one caregiver could very well be a source of satisfaction for another caregiver. Similarly, what a caregiver perceives to be stressful at one point might be perceived as pleasurable by that same caregiver under different circumstances. Just as caregivers' appraisals differ, we cannot assume that what works for one caregiver will necessary benefit another caregiver. Second, the inclusion of feedback arrows in the model in Figure 10.1 reminds us that caregiving is an ongoing process. As service providers, we must make sure that the timing of our interventions is appropriate. The dynamic nature of caregiving is such that both caregivers and the people for whom they care have changing needs. It is important to remember this, because a poorly timed intervention effort can do more harm than good to caregivers. A related issue is that changing any aspect of the caregiving situation will affect the rest of the system. Thus intervention efforts must be assessed for their impact throughout the system, in terms of both benefits and costs. Finally, the complexity of this model serves to remind us that the goal of helping caregivers is a large one, and that we must learn to be satisfied with small gains.

INTERVENTIONS INVOLVING
PATIENT-BASED STRESSORS

Obviously, the goal of any intervention is to enhance outcomes, either for the caregiver, the care recipient, or both (the caregiving dyad). Yet the target for the intervention typically is directed toward either the caregiver or the care recipient. With some notable exceptions (e.g., Quayhagen & Quayhagen, 1988), interventions to date have not targeted the caregiving dyad. And many interventions target the care recipient in an effort to reduce their caregiver's distress.

Interventions aimed at reducing primary caregiving stress (namely, aspects of the care recipient's condition) treat the care recipient as the primary target, yet seek to reduce the caregiver's distress. (Obviously, in the case of chronic illness, which often presents only limited potential for improvement, such interventions are not always feasible.) For example, use of medications and rehabilitative efforts might serve to make care recipients feel better, reduce their symptoms, improve their functioning, and reduce their need for care, resulting in increased independence. Intervention efforts aimed at these stressors often rely, at least to some extent, on the formal helping system.

While these interventions attempt to modify an aspect of the care recipient's illness, thereby reducing caregivers' primary stress, it is important to acknowledge the potential negative, as well as positive, affects the process of intervention can have on the caregiver. For example, interventions involving medication and rehabilitative efforts often require the caregiver's participation (e.g., administering medication, transporting care recipient to therapy, assisting with therapy "home work"). Thus, while the long-term benefits of such therapeutic efforts may be without question, it is important to consider potential demands of such interventions on caregivers.

It is also important to remember that interventions designed to improve an ailing care recipient's health have the potential to produce the positive, intended consequences but also can produce negative, unintended, consequences—for both caregiver and care recipient. For example, speech therapy for aphasia following a stroke can improve a care recipient's expressive and receptive skills and benefit the caregiver at the same time by restoring his or her ability to communicate with the care recipient. However, physical therapy for the same care recipient that results in increased mobility can be problematic if that person does not have the mental competence to refrain from engaging in potentially dangerous behaviors (e.g., wandering, self-injurious behavior).

The utility of interventions targeting aspects of the care recipient's impairment largely is determined by the type of impairment. For example, the rehabilitative efforts mentioned above are of far greater benefit to a person who has suffered a broken hip or a stroke than to someone with Alzheimer's disease. Thus, in identifying intervention efforts, it is necessary to take into account both the nature of the care recipient's impairment and the trajectory of recovery possible with that impairment as well as the potential benefits and costs (for a specific caregiver and care recipient) associated with the process and outcome of the specific intervention.

INTERVENTIONS INVOLVING CAREGIVER STRESS

Caregiver-based stressors typically include competing responsibilities between caregiving and other roles assumed by the caregiver (role-strain stressors). They also include stressful life events unrelated to caregiving that are experienced by the caregiver. Interventions aimed to reduce stress experienced by caregivers generally do so by diminishing the objective demands made upon them as caregivers through respite programs (Hooyman & Lustbader, 1986).

Respite programs range from formal day-care programs that allow caregivers to fulfill work or family responsibilities on a regular basis to informal arrangements that allow an alternative caregiver (e.g., another relative or friend) to relieve the major caregiver from responsibilities on special occasions. While such programs are extensively advocated, one must note that they are not always welcomed by recipients of help and sometimes result in greater burdens to caregivers when they resume caregiver tasks.

Respite programs can also benefit care recipients, if they offer well-supervised and successfully executed activities. Unintended consequences of such interventions, however, include extra expenses for caregivers and, often, feelings of guilt about leaving the care recipient in another's care. Potentially disruptive aspects of respite care have been illustrated in an investigation conducted by Berry and Zarit (1988). In an attempt to find out how caregivers who use respite services spend their time, caregivers were interviewed on days they used respite services and days that they did not use such services. Much to the researchers' surprise, results indicated that caregivers who used

day-care services, as opposed to in-home respite services, actually spent
more time with care recipients on the days that they had respite service. On
respite days, caregivers found themselves working even harder to ready the
care recipient for the service. This is just one example of how an intervention
(providing the caregiver with some free time) can potentially backfire.

INTERVENTIONS INVOLVING MEDIATORS

Given that, in many caregiving situations, the health of the care recipient
may not be readily improved (that is, primary stressors may not be modified),
and that mediating variables intervene between primary stressors and caregiving outcomes, many stress researchers have identified mediators as the
component of the stress process most amenable to successful intervention
(Gallagher, 1990; Pearlin, Turner, & Semple, 1989). Interventions aimed at
the second component of our model seek to provide the caregiver with
increase personal, social, or environmental resources.

While some intervention strategies aimed at caregiver-based stressors
may alter an objective aspect of the caregiving situation, others aim to reduce
stress by improving caregivers' appraisals concerning the objective, primary
stresses in caregiving. Interventions aimed at reducing a caregiver's intrapsychic strain include efforts to help them reappraise their caregiving situation by focusing on some of the uplifts in caregiving and to recognize,
articulate, and find ways to meet their needs. There are many strategies used
by formal and informal network members to help caregivers reappraise their
caregiving situation in a more positive light. Such interventions often rely on
informally boosting what we consider caregivers' coping resources, or out-
look. Rather than intervening to modify a care recipient's disability, interventions can target the caregiver's feelings concerning the objective stressors
in the model. The caregiver's emotions and feelings concerning the care
recipient's status might be modified through educational efforts or counseling sessions. Thus, for example, the wife of an elderly heart attack victim
who can no longer work may learn to focus on her husband's home skills
rather than his work-related skills as a source of pride and may learn to value
his contribution to the home. On the other hand, Johnson (1988) suggests that
caregivers may feel a sense of accomplishment and achievement at "taking
over" tasks that were previously assumed by the care recipient. For example,
a caregiving wife may take great pride in her newly acquired skills at
managing family finances. As with the interventions above, these efforts
could place added demands on an already burdened caregiver, or she may

face new responsibilities as challenges and appraise these challenges as an opportunity for growth.

Many caregivers report that support groups provide them with the important feeling that they are not alone. Just knowing that others are in a similar situation seems to help caregivers to reappraise their situation and conclude that things could be worse. We have yet to attend a support group meeting where a caregiver did not say, after sharing a particularly difficult caregiving event with the group, that "you have to laugh, or else you will cry." This refrain is met with understanding nods, faint chuckles, and, often, some creative suggestions for the problematic caregiving event. This scenario appears to help caregivers find humor in their situations and a sense of belonging.

In addition to managing their emotions regarding the feelings of hopelessness often reported by caregivers, some caregivers are able to appraise their caregiving situation more favorably when they conceptualize their role of caregiver as a profession. That is, many caregivers are able to be less critical of themselves, and their situation, when they are reminded that (a) caregiving is a job—often, more than a full-time job; (b) most caregivers never received training for the caregiving tasks they must assume; (c) most caregivers work seven days a week; and (d) many caregivers are so dedicated to their jobs that they never take any time off. Virtually all caregivers will report that they would not want to fly on an airplane piloted by someone who had never received flying lessons but who had, nonetheless, been flying the plane constantly for the past six days. This analogy frequently is more successful than the most impassioned plea in getting a caregiver to realize that he or she needs some "down time." (More formal interventions designed to foster increased resources are presented in the next section.) We anticipate that, in the future, interventions might similarly teach care recipients how to more effectively handle increased dependency brought about by an illness.

In addition to the mediating resource of appraisal, the most important personal resource available to a caregiver is his or her coping ability. The last two interventions discussed in the previous section loosely targeted caregivers' efforts to cope. Technically, coping refers to both behavioral and emotional strategies used by caregivers to deal with problematic encounters (Lazarus & Folkman, 1984). A variety of formal interventions attempt to increase caregivers' competence and ability to cope. (For a recent discussion of the value of coping for family caregivers and the importance of mediators on the stress-outcome link for caregivers, see Pearlin, Turner, & Semple, 1989.) These interventions are based on empirical data suggesting that people with lesser degrees of perceived competence tend to manage difficult events less successfully (Pagel, Becker, & Coppel, 1985). Among these interventions are those aimed at improving caregivers' assertiveness, enhancing their effectiveness at communicating with physicians and other formal health care providers, and increasing their personal coping resources (e.g., self-esteem).

A variety of therapeutic perspectives have been employed to boost caregivers' feelings of competence and ability to cope (e.g., Gallagher, Lovett, & Zeiss, 1989; Lovett & Gallagher, 1988; Zarit, in press). For example, Gallagher and associates direct an ongoing program of research at the Palo Alto, California, Veteran's Administration Hospital that is exploring the benefits of teaching caregivers to deal with their anger and depression, while Teri and colleagues (1990) at the University of Washington are similarly exploring the benefits of cognitive/behavior therapies as they relate to family caregivers. Regardless of the specific therapeutic approach, the underlying philosophy of these programs is that by enhancing caregivers' competence we are maximizing their abilities to deal with the stresses they encounter as caregivers.

Social supports, a second mediating resource, as indicated above, can come from either formal or informal helping network members and involves those exchanges where the caregiver receives informational or instrumental aid and/or affective/esteem support. This resource can have either the caregiver or care recipient as the primary target. The value of caregiving support groups, which directly target the caregiver, was discussed above. Yet research also suggests that support directly provided to the care recipient (e.g., friends and family members visiting with the care recipient) can also benefit the caregiver (Norris & Stephens, 1990; Zarit, Reever, & Bach-Peterson, 1980). An additional function of support groups and help from the formal network not mentioned above involves the exchange of information concerning relevant community services and programs.

A final goal for interventions aimed at mediators would be to increase caregivers' environmental resources. In this case, resources are defined broadly and can include financial aid and access to transportation, among others. An important set of interventions in this area relates to modification of the housing environments of frail elders, which, in turn, promotes independence in functioning and reduces dependence on caregivers.

INTERVENTIONS INVOLVING OUTCOMES

A final target for intervention within the proposed stress model is at the outcome stage. Outcomes in the model include caregivers' psychological and physical distress, and some interventions seek to intervene at this level.

Interventions aimed at reducing caregivers' psychological and physical distress include stress management programs; enhancing health through diet, exercise, and health promotion programs; and providing counseling and psychotherapy to reduce depression, anxiety, and other mental health symptomatology that can affect physical health. While some of these interventions are guided by the informal network, the formal helping system is more often the initiator of such intervention efforts.

Intervention at the outcome level should not be thought of as a "late" intervention. Although our simplified conceptual model does not show such feedback loops, such feedback in fact occurs from caregivers' outcomes back to primary stressors. Interventions at the outcome stage can be as effective as interventions aimed at primary or secondary stressors or their moderators.

From this discussion, it is apparent that caregivers typically are the primary target of intervention. With the exception of interventions aimed at modifying the objective primary stressor, most intervention strategies to date focus on only one member of the caregiving situation. One trend beginning to emerge in the caregiving stress literature is the exploration of the dyadic nature of caregiving situations. Recently, researchers at the Benjamin Rose Institute (e.g., Noelker & Townsend, 1988; Townsend & Noelker, 1988) have stressed the importance of considering the larger context in which caregiving occurs, and Quayhagen and Quayhagen (1988) have begun to explore interventions that target the caregiver-care-recipient dyad. Nonetheless, we need to expand further consideration of the dyadic nature of caregiving to include the family as a unit of analysis. Recent research conducted by Pruchno and her colleagues (1989) at the Philadelphia Geriatric Center suggests that, within caregiving families, no two members of the immediate family unit agree on the nature of the caregiving arrangement. While a discussion of this topic is beyond the scope of the present chapter, we anticipate that, in the future, interventions will target the larger caregiving unit, introducing even more complexity into an already complicated endeavor.

WHAT ARE WE OFFERING TO CAREGIVERS?

In an effort to address the diversity of caregiving situations and individual caregivers' needs, Rabins (1990) suggests three categories of interventions that might be of benefit to caregivers: (a) noble rhetoric, (b) education, and (c) resource availability. Noble rhetoric involves persuasion; it refers to any intervention that focuses on caregivers' perceptions and emotional states and provides them with understanding and emotional support. Education derives from learning theory and includes those interventions that result in behavior changes on the part of either the patient or the caregiver. Finally, resource availability is a pragmatic consideration: If caregivers perceive an adequate amount of resources to fulfill their caregiving responsibilities, it is possible that caregiving will not be perceived as stressful.

Based on the discussion above, interventions targeting certain components of the stress process can be categorized based on the function served by that intervention attempt. Interventions aimed at objective stressors tend to deal most frequently with resource availability and, to a lesser extent, education. On the other hand, interventions aimed at mediators and outcomes seem to serve the functions of noble rhetoric and education.

WHO HELPS?

Research on caregiving indicates that families and the informal helping network are responsible for the majority of assistance received by caregivers (Brody, 1981; Cantor, 1983; Stone, Cafferata, & Sangl, 1987) and that many caregivers turn to the formal helping network only when the informal network has been exhausted. Recent research efforts are beginning to examine the interface of informal and formal providers (e.g., Bass & Noelker, 1987; Chappel & Haven, 1985; Noelker & Townsend, 1987). Within the formal network are nonprofit agencies and commercial services. Falling between the informal and formal networks are self-help groups, which are more frequently used than the formal helping network. Results from investigations of the efficacy of various sources of interventions suggest that help, regardless of whether it comes from the formal or informal helping network, is equally effective (for a recent review, see Hattie, Sharpley, & Rogers, 1984).

WHERE DOES THE HELP OCCUR:
LOCATION OF THE INTERVENTION

Caregiving interventions occur in a variety of settings. Caregivers' needs for noble rhetoric typically are fulfilled by both the formal and informal networks and occur everywhere from the caregiver's home to a professional's office, and places in between. Resources such as respite and day-care services can occur in the caregiver's home or another site, and educational efforts usually occur outside the home. Location of an intervention is an important consideration in that it can serve to foster or impede a given caregiver's involvement in the intervention effort. It is the responsibility of the professional helper to acquaint himself or herself with the range of interventions to which caregivers are exposed and to help the caregiver identify those that are appropriate and those that are less than optimal.

TO INTERVENE OR NOT INTERVENE

Before undertaking a specific intervention within a particular caregiving situation, practitioners must consider whether the intervention is apt to facilitate the caregiving process (Rabins, 1990). Rabins points out that people who enter psychotherapy are clients identified by their distress; caregivers, however, often are thought to need help purely by virtue of the fact that they are caregivers. Within the caregiving stress literature, numerous empirical investigations have indicated that individuals' perceptions of events in caregiving, rather than the actual events themselves, are the best predictors of caregivers' distress (e.g., Haley, Brown, & Levine, 1987; Poulshock & Deimling, 1984; Zarit, in press, Zarit et al., 1980). These empirical results support clinical observations that, while some caregivers appear distressed, other caregivers seem to manage incredibly well. Thus we conclude that not all caregivers need help. Caregiving in and of itself is not synonymous with distress. Before introducing an intervention into a caregiving situation, need for such intervention, as well as the potential costs and benefits of the intervention, should be evaluated.

The importance of this point can be highlighted in a discussion of institutionalization. Clinical lore has long dictated that when the stresses of caregiving become excessive, institutionalization of the care recipient will serve to reduce caregivers' distress. Recent empirical investigations suggest, however, that caregiver stress often continues, and may even intensify, after institutionalization (e.g., George & Gwyther, 1984; Pagel, Becker, & Coppel, 1985; Pratt, Schmall, Wright, & Cleland, 1985). In an investigation comparing the stresses of in-home caregivers with caregivers to institutionalized care recipients, Kinney, Stephens, O'grocki, and Bridges (1989) found that, while caregivers to institutionalized care recipients reported fewer disruptions in their social lives, there were no differences between the two types of caregivers either in terms of depression or somatic symptoms. Regardless of where the care recipient resided, caregivers were equally bothered by care recipients' cognitive limitations and inappropriate behaviors. In summary, researchers examining institutionalization conclude that, while institutionalization may lessen the physical demands on caregivers, caregivers are faced with a new set of demands (e.g., relinquishing primary care responsibilities for the care recipient, interfacing with staff at the facility).

ALL CAREGIVERS ARE NOT ALIKE

Throughout our discussion, we have acknowledged the diversity of different caregiving situations. Consistent with this theme, Whitehouse (1990) recently stated that different caregivers have different expectations, that these expectations change over time, and that it is dangerous for health care providers to assume that they know what their clients want. This clinical observation is consistent with transactional models of stress that emphasize the importance of an individuals' appraisal, or interpretation, of an event in determining what is stressful. Research has amply documented that caregivers' subjective interpretation of caregiving tasks as stressful has a stronger impact on caregivers' well-being than the actual tasks themselves (Haley, Brown, & Levine, 1987; Kinney & Stephens, 1989b; Zarit et al., 1980).

Kinney and Stephens (1989a, 1989b) were interested in caregivers' perceptions of the daily caregiving stressors, or hassles, and the uplifts associated with caring for a demented family member. They adapted Lazarus and Folkman's conceptualization of chronic stress as hassles, or the minor events that are appraised by a caregiver as threatening his or her well-being. Lazarus and Folkman's conceptualization includes uplifts, or small satisfactions, as buffers against the negative accumulation of hassles. Kinney and Stephens generated a list of events that typically occur in caregiving (e.g., assisting the care recipient with eating, care recipient sleeping through the night, care recipient smiling). For each event that occurred during the past week, caregivers indicated how much of a hassle and/or an uplift that event was. Thus each event could be appraised (even by the same caregiver) as either a hassle or an uplift, both a hassle and an uplift, or neither a hassle nor a uplift.

Of interest to this discussion is the finding that of the 110 items, 84.5% were appraised by different caregivers as both hassles and uplifts. A total of 14.5% were appraised only as hassles, and one item was appraised only as an uplift. Thus more than four fifths of the caregiving events elicited both positive and negative appraisals by caregivers. These results indicate the importance of assessing caregivers' appraisals of events, because many of the same events were interpreted differently—that is, negatively and positively—by different respondents.

Examining individual caregivers' data from this study illustrates that even trained professionals need to exercise caution when deciding what their clients are experiencing. For example, several caregivers in the Kinney and Stephens study endorsed the item "care recipient sleeping through the night" to be a hassle, while they endorsed "extra expenses due to caregiving" to be an uplift. If you find this puzzling, consider the following: many caregivers reported that their care recipient typically stayed awake at night, watching television and wandering about the house. On those nights when the care recipient did not engage in their usual behavior, the caregiver stayed awake, wondering if the care recipient was ill. Meanwhile, the care recipient had a good night's sleep. The "hassle" came into play the next morning, when the caregiver, who had not slept well, if at all, had to supervise the care recipient, who had had his or her first good night's sleep in many days. Similarly, caregivers reported extra expenses associated with caregiving to be a blessing, because the "extra expenses" often meant that caregivers could afford some type of respite service. Empirical results such as these support recommendations by researchers (e.g., Lawton, Kleban, Moss, Rovine, & Glickspan, 1990; Stephens & Kinney, 1989) that caregivers' appraisals of events in caregiving are the key to learning about the stress process, and remind practitioners and researchers that frequently we do not know our clients/research participants as well as we thought.

MAKING THE SYSTEM MORE ACCESSIBLE

Having enumerated the valuable services provided by the formal sector, we must acknowledge a concern on our part. Recent evidence suggests that formal services tend to be under- rather than overutilized due to lack of availability of quality services, cost, transportation difficulties, and caregivers' feelings of guilt and anxiety over leaving their loved one in another's care (Brody, Saperstein, & Lawton, 1989). This is discouraging, in that the most enduring model of health care/service utilization (Andersen, 1968; Andersen & Newman, 1973) proposes that entry into the service system can be predicted by three factors: predisposing (demographic), enabling (availability), and need (subjective as well as objective) variables. The fact that caregivers, many of whom clearly need help, are not making use of available services suggests that a major challenge facing service providers is to facilitate caregivers' entry into the formal system.

In an attempt to understand this seeming contradiction, Gwyther (1990) has suggested that certain barriers prevent entry into the formal system and that, once in the formal system, caregivers' expectations often are not met. Gwyther maintains that most caregivers wait too long to enter the formal system, choosing instead to rely on the informal network until it reaches the point where it can no longer function. Upon entry into the formal system, many caregivers find that their needs are so great that they cannot be easily met. Gwyther suggests that practitioners might be in a position to encourage caregivers to make use of formal services earlier in the process so that their needs for control and continuity are more likely to be met. Given the dynamic nature of the caregiving process and the changing needs of both caregivers and care recipients, the timing of a given intervention becomes critical. In addition, Gwyther suggests that formal service providers should view families not as consumers but as clients who have both preferences and needs.

Consistent with Gwyther's belief that trust, rather than availability, leads to formal service utilization, Collins and her colleagues at Michigan State University (Collins, King, Stommel, Given, & Given, 1990) propose three sets of variables that influence family caregivers' intentions to seek services. These factors are classified as external cues to action (e.g., information, referral suggestion); caregiver and patient attitudes toward seeking help; and internal cues to action (e.g., caregivers' appraisals of the adequacy of informal supports, competency of supports, and their physical/psychological distress). These researchers conceptualize the role of a practitioner as a facilitator—a trained professional who, sensitive to the special demands faced by caregivers, can help them to negotiate and gain the maximum benefit from available services.

INTERVENTIONS: WHERE DO WE GO FROM HERE?

A current debate among researchers in the area of caregiving stress is whether we have over- or underestimated the extent to which caregiving is stressful. Some critics argue that stress researchers probably are more responsible for the creation of caregiving stress than are either caregivers or the recipients of their care. These critics suggest that researchers frequently find exactly what they look for; for example, if researchers set out to document how difficult caregiving is, they will not give up until they find stress among the respondents they study. Based on this reasoning, caregiving stress researchers have been challenged to consider the benefits to be gained from caring for a family member. Across a series of investigations, satisfactions in caregiving are being identified, and several researchers are suggesting that satisfactions in caregiving can, in fact, buffer the negative consequences of caregiving. While we are aware of the potential benefits of caring for a loved one, we also are aware of the potential difficulty such an arrangement can present.

Another concern with existing research on caregiving stress concerns issues of measurement. To date, the caregivers we have studied are a homogeneous group. Research participants typically are volunteers recruited from support groups; we know very little about non-support-group caregivers. Further, caregivers in most studies are white, middle class, and well educated. Current research such as that by Anderson (1990) and Segall and Wykle (1988), which focuses exclusively on minority caregivers and their experiences, will help to overcome our lack of knowledge in this area.

Currently, research on the utility of caregiving interventions is in its infancy stage. Research does, however, indicate that caregivers do need help, and social scientists are beginning to get a sense of how to help them. In a recent review of existing intervention studies, Zarit (1990) suggests that we have probably minimized the effectiveness of treatment strategies in several ways. First, Zarit maintains that the goals of our interventions have been too global and too ambitious. Given the stressful nature of caregiving, it is probably unrealistic to expect that our interventions can eliminate all of the pain associated with the decline of a loved individual that so many caregivers must endure. Oftentimes, too, professionals' goals do not match the caregivers' needs. For example, the stated goal of many day-care programs and respite services is to delay institutionalization. However, given the caregiving situations faced by many caregivers, delaying institutionalization may not be a realistic goal.

In focusing on interventions that occur to aid caregivers, our goal has been to provide an overview of different prototype interventions and place them within the organized conceptual framework of stress research. Rather than detailing the multitude of intervention strategies that have been reported, our goal was to provide a framework that can help clinicians identify caregiver needs that call for intervention and tailor intervention strategies to those needs. A flexible framework that allows clinicians to target interventions to areas of maximum cost/benefit may be found useful in considering unique aspects of each caregiver's situation. Understanding observed regularities in the caregiving paradigm can offer guidelines for such intervention strategies. Our hope is that researchers and practitioners may adapt and modify the framework presented to make them relevant to the specific caregiving situations they are addressing.

In the process of outlining a conceptual framework, we inevitably note the many gaps in knowledge and many conceptual ambiguities that characterize our current understanding of the caregiving process. We also are reminded of the complexities that challenge both researchers and practitioners in designing, targeting, and implementing caregiving interventions. Each new element of this complexity, once it has been identified and described, represents an added opportunity for designing innovative programs that will be effective in assisting those engaged in assisting others. Ultimately, a conceptual model may be developed that allows practitioners to determine with some confidence (a) whether intervention is necessary; (b) what aspect of the caregiving situation should be modified; (c) what type of intervention is most likely to be effective; (d) who should intervene; (e) when is the appropriate time for intervention; and (f) the likely consequences of intervention, both positive and negative.

REFERENCES

Andersen, R. (1968). *A behavioral model of families' use of health services.* Chicago: Center for Health Administration Studies.

Andersen, R., & Newman, J. (1973). Societal and individual determinants of medical care utilization in the United States. *Milbank Memorial Fund Quarterly, 51,* 95-124.

Anderson, N. (1990, March). *Mental and physical health in minority caregivers.* Paper presented at the National Institute of Mental Health workshops on the Mental Health of Family Caregivers in Alzheimer's Disease and Related Dementias, Washington, DC.

Anthony-Bergstone, C., Zarit, S. H., & Gatz, M. (1988). Symptoms of psychological distress among caregivers of dementia patients. *Psychology and Aging, 3,* 245-248.

Bass, D. M., & Noelker, L. S. (1987). The influence of family caregivers on elders' use of in-home services: An expanded conceptual model. *Journal of Health and Social Behavior, 28,* 184-196.

Berry, G. L., & Zarit, S. H. (1988, November). *Caregivers' activities on respite and non-respite days: A comparison of two service approaches.* Paper presented at the annual meeting of the Gerontological Society of America, San Francisco.

Biegel, D. E., & Blum, A. (Eds.). (1988-1989). Aging and family caregivers [Special issue]. *Journal of Applied Social Sciences, 13.*

Brody, E. M. (1981). Women in the middle and family help to older people. *The Gerontologist, 21,* 471-480.

Cantor, M. H. (1983). Strain among caregivers: A study of experience in the United States. *The Gerontologist, 23,* 597-604.

Chappel, N. L., & Haven, B. (1985). Who helps the elderly person: A discussion of informal and formal care. In W. A. Peterson & J. Quadagno (Eds.), *Social bonds in later life.* Beverly Hills, CA: Sage.

Collins, C., King, S., Stommel, M., Given, C. W., & Given, B. (1990, March). Service utilization by dementia caregivers. Paper presented at the National Institute of Mental Health workshops on the Mental Health of Family Caregivers in Alzheimer's Disease and Related Dementias, Washington, DC.

Danis, B. G. (1978, November). *Stress in individuals caring for ill elderly relatives.* Paper presented at the annual meeting of the Gerontological Society of America, Dallas, TX.

Gallagher, D. (1990, March). *Depression-oriented versus anger-oriented therapies.* Paper presented at the National Institute of Mental Health workshops on the Mental Health of Family Caregivers in Alzheimer's Disease and Related Dementias, Washington, DC.

Gallagher, D., Lovett, S., & Zeiss, A. (1989). Interventions with caregivers of frail elderly persons. In M. Ory & K. Bond (Eds.), Aging and health care: Social science and policy perspectives (pp. 167-190). London: Routledge & Kegan Paul.

George, & Gwyther, L. (1984, November). *The dynamics of caregiver burden: Changes in caregiver well-being over time.* Paper presented at the annual meeting of the Gerontological Society of America, San Antonio, TX.

Gwyther, L. (1990, March). Paper presented at the National Institute of Mental Health workshops on the Mental Health of Family Caregivers in Alzheimer's Disease and Related Dementias, Washington, DC.

Haley, W. E., Brown, S. L., & Levine, E. G. (1987). Family caregiver appraisals of patient behavioral disturbances in senile dementia. *Clinical Gerontologist, 6,* 25-34.

Hattie, J. H., Sharpley, C. F., & Rogers, H. J. (1984). Comparative effectiveness of professional and paraprofessional helpers. *Psychological Bulletin, 95,* 534-541.

Hooyman, N. R., & Lustbader, W. (1986). *Taking care of your aging family members: A practical guide.* New York: Free Press.

Johnson, C. L. (1988). Relationships among family members and friends in later life. In R. M. Milardo (Ed.), *Families and social networks* (pp. 168-189). Newbury Park, CA: Sage.

Kahana, B., & Kahana, E. (1984). Stress reactions. In P. Lewinsohn & L. Teri (Eds.), *Clinical Geropsychology* (pp. 139-169). New York: Pergamon.

Kahana, E., Kahana, B., & Young, R. (1987). Strategies of coping and post-institutional outcomes. *Research on Aging, 9,* 182-199.

Kahana, E., & Young, R. (1990). Clarifying the caregiver paradigm: Challenges for the future. In D. E. Biegel & A. Blum (Eds.), *Aging and caregiving: Theory, research and policy* (pp. 76-97). Newbury Park, CA: Sage.

Kinney, J. M., & Stephens, M.A.P. (1989a). Caregiving hassles scale: Assessing the daily hassles of caring for a family member with dementia. *The Gerontologist, 29,* 328-332.

Kinney, J. M., & Stephens, M.A.P. (1989b). Hassles and uplifts of giving care to a family member with dementia. *Psychology and Aging, 4,* 402-408.

Kinney, J. M., Stephens, M.A.P., O'grocki, P. K., & Bridges, A. M. (1989, November). *Hassles and well-being among AD caregivers: The in-home versus institutional experience.* Paper presented at the annual meeting of the Gerontological Society of America, Minneapolis, MN.

Lawton, M. P., Kleban, M. H., Moss, M. Rovine, M., & Glickspan, A. (1989). Measuring caregiving appraisal. *Journal of Gerontology: Psychological Sciences, 44,* 61-71.

Lazarus, R. S., & Folkman, S. (1984). *Stress, appraisal, and coping.* New York: Springer.

Lovett, S., & Gallagher, D. (1988). Psychoeducational interventions for family caregivers: Preliminary efficacy date. *Behavior Therapy, 19,* 331-344.

Moss, M., Lawton, M. P., Dean J., Goodman, M., & Schneider, J. (1987, November). *Satisfactions and burdens in caring for impaired elderly persons.* Paper presented at the annual meeting of the Gerontological Society of America, Washington, DC.

Norris, V. K., & Stephens, M.A.P. (1990). Submitted for presentation at the annual meeting of the Gerontological Society of America, Boston: November.

Noelker, L. S., & Townsend, A. L. (1987). Perceived caregiving effectiveness: The impact of parental impairment, community resources, and caregiver characteristics. In T. Brubaker (Ed.), *Aging, health, and family: Long-term care* (pp. 58-79). Newbury Park, CA: Sage.

Pagel, M. D., Becker, J., & Coppel, D. B. (1985). Loss of control, self-blame, and depression: An investigation of spouse caregivers of Alzheimer's disease patients. *Journal of Abnormal Psychology, 94,* 169-182.

Pearlin, L. T. (1983). Role strains and personal stress. In H. B. Kaplan (Ed.), *Psychosocial stress: Trends in research and theory.* NY: Academic Press.

Pearlin, L. I., Turner, H., & Semple, S. (1989). Coping and the mediation of caregiver stress. In E. Light & B. D. Lebowitz (Eds.), *Alzheimer's disease, treatment and family stress: Directions for research* (pp. 198-217). Washington, DC: U.S. Department of Health and Human Services.

Poulshock, W. S., & Deimling, G. T. (1984). Families caring for elders in residence: Issues in the measurement of burden. *Journal of Gerontology, 39,* 230-239.

Pratt, C. C., Schmall, V. L., Wright, S., & Cleland, M. (1985). Burden and coping strategies of caregivers to Alzheimer's patients. *Family Relations, 34,* 27-33.

Pruchno, R. (1989). Alzheimer's disease and families: Methodological advances. In E. Light & B. D. Lebowitz (Eds.), *Alzheimer's disease, treatment and family stress: Directions for research* (pp. 174-195). Washington, DC: U.S. Department of Health and Human Services.

Quayhagen, M. P., & Quayhagen, M. (1988). Alzheimer's stress: Coping with the caregiving role. *The Gerontologist, 28,* 391-396.

Rabins, P. (1990, March). *Clinical interventions with Alzheimer caregivers.* Paper presented at the National Institute of Mental Health workshops on the Mental Health of Family Caregivers in Alzheimer's Disease and Related Dementias, Washington, DC.

Schulz, R. (1990, March). *What is the scope of the problem? Evidence on mental and physical morbidity in Alzheimer caregivers.* Paper presented at the National Institute of Mental Health workshops on the Mental Health of Family Caregivers in Alzheimer's Disease and Related Dementias, Washington, DC.

Seelbach, W. C. (1978). Correlates of aged parents filial responsibility, expectation, and realizations. *Family Coordinator, 27,* 341-350.

Segall, M., & Wykle, M. (1988). The black family's experience with dementia. *Journal of Applied Social Sciences, 13,* 170-191.

Stephens, M.A.P., & Kinney, J. M. (1989). Caregiving stress instruments: Assessment of content and measurement quality. *Gerontology Review, 2,* 40-54.

Stone, R., Cafferata, G. L., & Sangl, J. (1987). Caregivers of the frail elderly: A national profile. *The Gerontologist, 27,* 616-626.

Teri, L. (1990, March). *Behavioral treatment of depression in dementia patients: The role of the family caregiver.* Paper presented at the National Institute of Mental Health workshops on the Mental Health of Family Caregivers in Alzheimer's Disease and Related Dementias, Washington, DC.

Toseland, R. W., & Smith, G. C. (in press). Supporting family caregivers of the frail elderly. In A. Gitterman (Ed.), *Handbook of social work practice with people in oppressive life circumstances.* New York: Columbia University Press.

Townsend, A. L., & Noelker, L. S. (1987). The impact of family relationships on perceived caregiving effectiveness. In T. Brubaker (Eds.), *Aging, health, and family: Long-term care* (pp. 80-99). Newbury Park, CA: Sage.

Whitehouse, P. J. (1990). *Special challenges in research on the mental health/physical health interface in caregivers: Future directions.* Paper presented at the National Institute of Mental Health workshops on the Mental Health of Family Caregivers in Alzheimer's Disease and Related Dementias, Washington, DC.

Young, R., & Kahana, E. (1987). Conceptualizing stress, coping, and illness management in heart disease caregiving. *The Hospice Journal, 3.*

Zarit, S. H. (1990). Do we need another study on caregiving? *The Gerontologist,*

Zarit, S. H. (in press). Interventions with frail elders and their families: Are they effective and why? In M.A.P. Stephens, J. H. Crowther, S. Hobfall, & D. Tennenbaum (Eds.), *Stress and coping in late life families.* Washington, DC: Hemisphere.

Zarit, S. H., Orr, N. K., & Zarit, J. M. (1985). *The hidden victims of Alzheimer's disease: Families under stress.* New York: New York University Press.

Zarit, S. H., Reever, K., & Bach-Peterson, J. (1980). Relatives of the impaired elderly: Correlates of feelings of burden. *The Gerontologist, 20,* 649-655.

Chapter 11

INTERVENTION STRATEGIES
Support Services for Family Caregivers

LEON SCHRAUBEN

As our society ages, the number of older adults with chronic disease and functional limitations also increases, creating a situation where many older people need some form of assistance to maintain their independence. This assistance or caregiving is provided largely by family members, many of whom do not feel adequately prepared and informed regarding the services that may be available to help them. Caregivers most often are female spouses and adult children who have numerous family, work, and social responsibilities in addition to caring for their elderly, functionally impaired relative. These caregivers look to human service agencies and health care providers for information and guidance to carry out their responsibilities.

Health care providers usually cannot manage the care of older people presenting with multiple chronic diseases and several dependencies in activities of daily living in isolation, but rather they require a coordination of services with many community agencies to assist the patient and caregiver. Collaboration, interdisciplinary assessment, and case management are significant strategies for health care providers to better serve this population.

THE FRAIL ELDERLY

Older people experiencing a decline in function and requiring assistance from another person to perform personal care activities and home management activities (often referred to as activities of daily living and instrumental activities of daily living) can be described as "the frail elderly." For these people, independence often hinges on the availability of family and others to assist with daily chores or personal care needs. Delay, disruption, or cancellation of services ultimately may have catastrophic effects leading to institutionalization for the older person with functional limitations.

When bathing, dressing, eating, transferring, walking, getting outside, and using the toilet were assessed in the National Health Interview Survey (National Center for Health Statistics [NCHS], 1987) 10% of noninstitutionalized people age 65 and older reported receiving assistance with at least one personal care activity. Nearly 3% reported receiving assistance with four to seven personal care activities. For those 85 years and older, more than 30% reported having at least one care activity for which they receive help, while over 10% received help with four to seven personal care activities. Bathing, getting outside, and dressing were the most commonly cited activities requiring assistance.

Home management activities such as preparing meals, dressing, managing money, using the telephone, doing heavy housework, and doing light housework also were assessed through self-reporting, with over 20% of the noninstitutionalized elderly stating that they receive assistance with at least one home management activity (NCHS, 1987), and 5% reporting that they receive assistance with four to six home management activities. Over 50% of people age 85 and older report receiving help with at least one of these activities, while 22% receive assistance with four to six home management activities. Doing heavy housework and shopping were the most common activities for which older people were dependent on family and others for assistance.

The frail elderly can be further defined in terms of mental status. Certainly cognitive impairment affects the older person's ability to perform activities of daily living and home management. It is conservatively estimated that 10% to 15% of people 65 years of age and older are suffering with mild, moderate, or severe dementia, while 25% of the over-85 population is estimated to have dementia (Michigan Department of Public Health, 1987). The majority of these dementing diseases are irreversible and progressive, increasing the personal care and home management needs of the person afflicted and adding stress to an already overextended family caregiver.

Aging increases the risk of cognitive impairment and functional limitations. Advanced aging increases the likelihood of experiencing functional impairment in multiple areas of personal care and home management. The old-old, those 85 years of age and older, are the most at risk of losing their independence without the support of their caregivers.

CAREGIVERS

Spouses and adult children are the most frequent providers of assistance with activities of daily living when help is needed. The older spouse-caregiver is a particular target for intervention services. In a survey of Michigan residents age 60 and older (Michigan Office of Services to the Aging, 1987) 11% reported that they were providing care for one or more persons in their home because of injury, disability, or long-term illness. Over 40% of those receiving care from an older person were husbands or wives, 20% were aged parents, and 11% were siblings. The remaining were children, friends, or other relatives. Furthermore, over 16% of those elderly providing care for others with functional limitations were assisting two to five people.

Few people have any advanced training in caregiving or choose it as a role for themselves in the context of their family. They often do not anticipate caregiving or desire the situation to continue. Although most caregivers are female and provide 80% to 90% of the assistance with bathing and dressing the functionally limited adult, their caregiving responsibilities vary a great deal and change unexpectedly (Michigan Office of Services to the Aging, 1987). This unpredictable progression in caregiving is difficult to plan for. At best a caregiver can anticipate a range of problems his or her loved one may experience but probably will not be able to plan for their sequence or severity. Caregiving responsibilities can have a major impact upon personal, marital, work, and family life.

For adult children, caregiving may take its greatest toll on the caregiver's emotional status. Over 50% report a change for the worse in their general emotional state (Horowitz, 1982). In addition, 47% report less time available for recreation and leisure activities; 36% feel their plans for the future (including job changes, relocation, and retirement) have changed for the worse; 33% report a decline in physical health and stamina, while the same percentage also has difficulty relaxing and sleeping. Significantly for adult children caregivers experiencing a change in how close they feel to their parent, this change is for the better by more than a 4 to 1 margin. A majority, however, report no change in how close they feel to their parent, and the close feeling some have does not translate into getting along better with their parent.

In summary, caregivers predominately are females taking on a responsibility that is difficult to manage in the face of numerous personal, work, and family responsibilities. It is not a job they seek out or for which they feel adequately prepared. Caregiving significantly affects all areas of the person's life, including their sense of physical and emotional well-being.

COMMUNITY RESOURCES

Caregivers use community resources to assist in maintaining the impaired elderly in the least restrictive environment and to avoid institutionalization. Resources can be used to further evaluate the functionally limited older person, assist in direct care in the home, provide quality social interaction and support for caregivers, and to provide legal and financial assistance as well. Use of community resources can be viewed in terms of the progression of services required as caregiving needs increase and intensify. Much variety exists in the availability of services and how they are delivered from state to state and community to community.

Three agencies that are very helpful and exist for every community are Area Agencies on Aging, Department of Social Services, and Community Mental Health Boards. The Area Agency on Aging is the federally mandated agency charged with coordinating national and state programs serving the elderly. In addition, Social Service Departments and Community Mental Health agencies provide a number of services for older adults and frequently have specialized programs in administering them. These agencies can be a starting point in discovering what is available in the community.

HEALTH CARE SERVICES FOR THE IMPAIRED ELDER

Geriatric assessment centers exist in many communities and their numbers are increasing. Health, mental health, and human service professionals specializing in geriatrics and gerontology join together in an interdisciplinary team to assess a person's physical, mental, functional, social, financial, and environmental status to ensure a comprehensive evaluation. Geriatric assessment centers often differ in their design and staffing, methods of collecting data, and focus of evaluation. Therefore there is wide variability in their scope and intensity. Common goals include provision of a comprehensive assessment of a person's functional status, education for patient and family regarding the cause of any functional limitations, and recommendations of community services that could assist the family in caregiving.

Acute care facilities and primary care clinics are used in much the same way as with other populations; however, the frequency of use and care of people with multiple health problems are significant characteristics that might indicate the need for a consultation with a physician specializing in geriatric medicine. Geriatricians are available in many areas and have specialized knowledge of the aging process utilized for consultation or primary care responsibilities.

In-home health agencies provide a variety of services and exist in most communities. Physical, occupational, and speech therapists, nurses, medical social workers, nutritionists, and home health aides usually are available in these agencies. A physician's referral is required for their services, which can include skilled nursing care, health assessments, education, coordination of home services, rehabilitative therapy, health and mental health counseling, nutrition assessment and counseling, general hygiene assistance, meal preparation, and referral to other community services as needed. In-home nursing agencies require short-term, rehabilitative care to be covered by Medicare. Custodial, general maintenance care needed by functionally limited older adults is usually not covered by Medicare for any length of time.

Mental health services are provided by most community mental health agencies on an outpatient basis; however, many are now offering outreach counseling to functionally limited older adults in the home. These services are usually provided by individuals possessing a master's degree in social work with special training in gerontology and include short-term mental health counseling, substance abuse and alcohol counseling, and nursing home consultation. Case management of clients to coordinate resources also may be available. As noted, medical social workers provide short-term counseling through in-home nursing agencies for those people having this service. In addition, many psychiatrists, psychologists, and psychiatric social workers are now specializing in the unique needs of the frail elderly and their caregivers. Unfortunately, most have been unable to implement an outreach component in their practice and require that the person be seen as an outpatient. Inpatient geropsychiatry programs exist in many communities and may be helpful in treating the person with more acute psychiatric problems.

Specialized services exist including dental, vision, and hearing evaluation programs. Additionally, health clinics such as nursing clinics and foot clinics may be very helpful in meeting the health care needs of this population.

Nutrition services also are available. Congregate meal sites often are located at senior centers and day programs for the cognitively and functionally impaired. For persons who would have great difficulty in getting to a meal site, home-delivered meals are an excellent source of nutrition and, in addition, may provide the elderly person with social contact. Congregate and home-delivered meal programs frequently are coordinated by the local Area Agency on Aging in addition to other community agencies. Food stamps and government surplus food programs also are available to the functionally impaired elderly with limited incomes. The Department of Social Services administers the food stamp program, and surplus foods are coordinated from a variety of community agencies. Food banks exist in most medium-size and larger American cities to assist low-income persons with food needs and emergency situations.

OTHER SERVICES

Senior centers exist in most areas and provide a variety of social activities to their participants. Often other community services are associated with them such as transportation programs and congregate meals. Senior centers can be a resource for the functionally limited older adult in areas where day programs for cognitively and functionally impaired elderly do not exist. Many senior centers in these areas work well with participants experiencing a wide range of functional ability. Also, senior centers may be the first option for social activity for those persons moderately limited, as some day programs cater to the person with advanced impairment.

Transportation services vary a great deal; however, most areas have some type of subsidized program for the elderly such as reduced-fee taxi service, accessible lift vans, or volunteer care drivers. Often services are restricted to certain hours of the day and, in rural areas, specified days of the week. As noted previously, many day programs provide their own transportation in limited areas. Unaccompanied people with cognitive impairment frequently are limited in their ability to use transportation services, as most programs do not provide supervision or companionship. Wheelchair users also are often without transportation due to the lack of accessible vans or assistance in transferring to an automobile.

Legal services are available to the elderly in many areas at reduced cost or free. Consultation with a lawyer knowledgeable in the law as it affects older people with functional limitations is important in addressing issues of competency and guardianship. Transfer of assets to spouses and family members affects eligibility for Medicaid and Supplemental Security Income. Income support programs vary from state to state in terms of their eligibility requirements and services they reimburse. The Area Agency on Aging may be helpful in identifying legal services available.

Homemaker services frequently are available to the frail, low-income elderly from the Department of Social Services and Area Agency on Aging. Services vary greatly and can range from 20 hours per week, to home maintenance assistance, to one visit every two weeks to do laundry, light housekeeping, and grocery shopping. Sometimes programs exist with sliding fee scales. Homemaker services also are usually offered by in-home nursing agencies for an hourly fee.

Companionship and response services can be very helpful. Many community agencies and religious groups provide companionship and friendly visiting. These services provide the functionally limited person with quality social interaction perhaps unrelated to care needs. This is a significant factor in that the elderly impaired person has a need to respond to people other than in the sick role.

Alert/response systems are those services through which an impaired older adult can be monitored to detect any changes in his or her environment to allow for direct communication to health care providers in cases of emergency. The *Carrier Alert Program,* an example of an alert service, allows for the postal carrier or an intermediary to contact family or friends of an aged person if the carrier suspects something is wrong in the home. Mail carriers can be well-informed regarding the usual routine of residents on their route and may notice uncharacteristic changes before family or friends call on the person. Response systems such as *Lifeline* allow the at-risk elderly to push a button to receive assistance from a local emergency service or health care agency. The emergency service has pertinent data on file regarding the person's medical status and people identified to check in on the patient when the system is activated. If no one can be located to check in on the person, a health care provider is sent to assess the situation. Alert/response systems offer peace of mind to persons receiving the service and their caregivers.

HOUSING OPTIONS

Housing options are numerous for the functionally limited elderly and vary a great deal with geographic area. In-home supported programs, subsidized housing, and perhaps retirement communities exist in most medium-size and larger communities, while adult foster care may not exist at all in some areas. Additionally, housing options are called by different names from state to state, and services provided will vary due to regulating restrictions.

In-home services to assist the person either in his or her own home or in a relative's home most frequently are the first option identified by family. Independence and maintenance of a home are strong values in our society. Persons with mild to moderate impairment often can be assisted in maintaining their independence with monitoring and coordinating by their family caregiver. Progression in limitations may make other living arrangements more desirable when supervision and direct care needs increase.

Shared housing arrangements often are initiated voluntarily; however, some areas now have formal programs to interview and match prospective boarders with householders. Unique agreements are forged based upon the householders' needs and the boarders' abilities. Most shared housing arrangements exclude direct personal care, focusing on companionship, structured routine, and household chores as services to be provided by the boarder. These services are negotiated for room and board, at times with no money changing hands. Some programs match older adults with their peers, while others emphasize intergenerational relationships. Shared housing programs work well with moderately impaired householders and couples where there is an elderly caregiver to an impaired spouse. They also seem to flourish in areas where there is a housing shortage and in university neighborhoods.

Congregate living arrangements are called by various names in places where they exist, with the same name used by states to designate different classifications of services. Residents have private or semiprivate rooms with shared common areas. Meals usually are prepared for the house, and transportation may be provided. Collective activities and housecleaning services often are available. Congregate living arrangements vary in number of residents from region to region.

Senior housing is most often characterized by efficiency or one-bedroom apartments for the elderly with little to no supervision; usually a variety of voluntary activities and congregate meals are available. Senior housing units often are subsidized by federal, state, or local governments and in some areas provide an excellent housing option for socially isolated older adults, people with moderate incomes, and the elderly with less inhibiting functional limitations.

Adult foster care homes or personal care homes usually provide 24-hour supervision, administer oral medications, provide housecleaning and laundry services, prepare meals, and assist in transportation for health care appointments. Adult foster care homes are an excellent housing resource when

24-hour supervision becomes necessary yet nursing care is not required. They delay, sometimes indefinitely, the need for institutionalization and usually cost about one third to one half of what nursing homes require. The adult foster care home is usually small (consisting of perhaps 4 to 10 residents) and frequently is the residence of the proprietor, creating a very homelike atmosphere. In some areas, assistance with bathing, dressing, toileting, and other activities of daily living are provided. Some states have reimbursement programs to assist low-income persons with foster care payment.

Life care communities or continuing care communities provide a variety of care levels on one campus. Usually, independent apartments, personal care programs, and skilled nursing facilities exist in one development, sometimes consisting of separate buildings or different wings or floors. The goal of continuing care communities is to meet the changing needs of the older adult in one setting. In some housing developments the skilled nursing component is not available; in others, only the intermediate-level, personal care service is provided. Often these limited communities are called luxury senior housing--luxurious in the services they provide. Continuing care communities often can require a significant entry fee or down payment in addition to a monthly fee. They provide an excellent housing alternative for the well elderly and those moderately impaired in terms of the security they provide on one campus.

SUPPORT FOR CAREGIVERS

Perhaps nothing else is of more significance in maintaining family caregiving than services in support of the caregiver. Several programs exist that provide free time or respite care and education and emotional support to family caregivers. Such programs enable caregivers to maintain their assistance to the functionally limited relative.

Respite care is scheduled time free from responsibilities for the primary caregiver to tend to other personal, family, work, or recreational activities in addition to an opportunity to rest and recoup energies. Respite care includes in-home services as well as inpatient programs. It can be an afternoon per week in one's own home or a two-week stay in an inpatient respite program enabling the family to take a vacation. Inpatient respite programs are scarce in many areas but seem to be increasing in number. Innovative programs are developing in association with hospitals, nursing facilities, and adult foster care homes. These services often are not covered by Medicare or other insurance and can be expensive. Respite care services in the home can be arranged with in-home nursing agencies and independent aides in addition to utilizing the volunteer efforts of neighbors, friends, and other family members for scheduled time free of responsibilities for the primary caregiver. Many community agencies are developing specific respite programs, training volunteers to provide this service for free, or using sliding fee scales. The local Area Agency on Aging would be the first place to explore respite options available in the community.

Day programs for the mentally impaired and functionally limited elderly provide further respite service for the caregiver while giving quality social-ization and stimulation time for the older person. These programs frequently operate 5 days per week, 6 to 8 hours per day, and often provide transportation for their participants. Day programs attempt to offer interesting activities developed specifically for the impaired older adult while taking care not to frustrate or overstimulate them. The benefit to caregiver and participant can be significant in improving the quality of life for both and, in doing so, can delay, sometimes indefinitely, institutionalization.

Support groups for caregivers abound and appear to be increasing in number. The Alzheimer's Association, formerly Alzheimer's Disease and Related Disorders Association (ADRDA), has been instrumental in develop-ing and maintaining support groups for caregivers of persons with dementia. Caregiver support groups also are often associated with other specific dis-eases, such as Huntington's or Parkinson's diseases, and are frequently sponsored by day programs, social service, mental health, aging, and health organizations. Support groups can be ongoing or closed-ended in time and many, especially the short-term groups, have strong educational components in addition to providing emotional support and guidance by those experienc-ing similar problems. The various groups associated with illnesses and national organizations publish a great deal of helpful information for care-givers, the general public, and professionals alike. Many groups focus on specific caregiving populations, for example, spouse, adult children, or a day-program participant group for family members.

Inpatient and home care hospice programs can be helpful for families caring for someone with an identifiable short-term prognosis, usually six months or less. Many people with functional limitations due to chronic progressive disease do not fill this requirement. The general progression of disease can be anticipated; however, time frames may be difficult or impos-sible to identify.

Employee assistance programs, available to many American workers, often assist with information and referral for problems in the employee's family. Unique agencies, such as Work/Family Elder Directions of Massachusetts, have developed information and referral programs independently, contracting with larger companies to provide this service as a benefit to their employees. It is increasingly recognized that caregiving responsibilities can be a factor influencing job performance, so innovative employers are addressing this need.

COLLABORATION

The key to effective assessment of needs in the functionally impaired elderly, and identification and management of services to assist in meeting these needs for families as well as impaired elders, is the collaboration of health and human service care providers in the community. Rarely can a single agency or service provider work in isolation to comprehensively meet needs.

Collaboration is more than making referrals to community agencies or providing families with program phone numbers; it is engaging other agencies and disciplines in the assessment process. The frail elderly present with problems too complex to fully access in a clinic appointment or intake interview, and the task at hand may not be best handled by that particular professional. The knowledge and skills of professionals available should dictate who addresses a particular problem. Good communication is essential to effective collaboration in geriatric care.

INTERDISCIPLINARY AND MULTIDISCIPLINARY GERIATRIC ASSESSMENT

Takamura (1983) distinguishes between multidisciplinary and interdisciplinary assessment by, among other things, assessing the group's goals—collective versus individual. An interdisciplinary team is composed of a mix of professionals from various backgrounds, such as a physician, nurse, and social worker, joining together to form an identity as a collective unit. The unit is more important than the individual disciplines, and goals are identified by the team rather than by individual members. Multidisciplinary teams are also composed of various disciplines; however, the individual profession is more important than the collective identification. Goals usually are individual, with team members sharing information versus working interdependently. The highest ranking professional on the team is usually the one taking a leadership role. It is important to note the differences between multidisciplinary and interdisciplinary teams, when involved in collaborative efforts, to ensure that all members are operating under similar assumptions regarding process and outcome.

The rationale for interdisciplinary geriatric assessment includes the complex nature of problems experienced by older adults with functional impairment and the inherent diverse nature of gerontology. As discussed earlier, the functionally limited person experiences an interaction of physical, psychological, social, economic, and environmental factors coming together to form a profile of characteristics to be assessed comprehensively. Diverse professions have developed gerontological foci specializing in the needs of older people within the context of their professional scope of practice.

The frail elderly benefit the most from interdisciplinary assessment. People with multiple medical and psychosocial problems presenting with limited support systems and experiencing a decline in function with perhaps several dependencies in activities of daily living are better served by a comprehensive, collaborative effort. Persons with uncertain etiology of dementia benefit from interdisciplinary assessment and usually fit the profile described.

The goals of interdisciplinary geriatric assessment (Baldwin & Tsukuda, 1981) include (a) development of long-term care plans; (b) maintenance and improvement of functional independence; (c) promotion of the appropriate and efficient use of community services; (d) maintenance of the impaired person in the least restrictive environment; and (e) addressing the issue of caregiver stress.

Principles of effective team functioning (Given & Simmons, 1977; Margolis & Fiorell, 1984) include collaboration and collegiality; clear communication; coordination of services or case management; common goal setting; team accountability for patient outcomes; stability; productive conflict resolution; and compromise and negotiation. Barriers to effective team functioning include territoriality or "turf" issues; control, competitive, and professional dominance issues; role conflict; ineffective decision making and problem solving; nonproductive conflict; unclear, inconsistent team process; and lack of coordination of services within the team.

Multidisciplinary teams have similar effective principles and barriers to team functioning with the exception of common goals replaced by individual professional goals. Team functioning operates in the structure of hierarchical professional status or with a clearly identified leader coordinating individual efforts. Multidisciplinary geriatric assessment works well when professionals from diverse community agencies come together to collaborate on a specific case or develop an interagency protocol for assessment of the functionally limited elderly.

For both styles of geriatric assessment, Baldwin and Tsukuda (1981) identify general advantages for professionals in collaboration. These include availability of a greater range of knowledge, skills, and services; greater efficiency through coordination and integration of services; increased communication and support among providers; and greater opportunity to practice at the highest level of skill and training.

CASE MANAGEMENT

Case management strategies are given much attention at present yet are not new at all, being part of original social casework theory in social work and typical of nurses' responsibilities in a hospital. Primary physicians may manage health care consultations and referrals but usually do not coordinate social service resources for their patients.

Case management can be defined as coordination of a comprehensive, multidimensional assessment; developing care plans and recommendations; monitoring services and reassessing needs; and responsibility for coordination by a single team or person (Kane, 1988). Case management teams in many settings are composed of a nurse and social worker working together to coordinate assessment and monitor services. Implementing an informal team process and long-term planning are principles of case management. The rationale for case management is similar to that of interdisciplinary geriatric assessment in that it addresses the complex needs of the functionally limited elderly in a vast, confusing service delivery room. Its goals are to coordinate assessment and monitor services in the least restrictive environment for the frail elderly at risk of institutionalization.

In a framework of case management, systems can be open or closed (White & Simmons, 1988) depending on their target population. Recipients of case management can be clients of a larger structure such as a health care or social service organization or nonclient, community residents contracting only for case management services. A health care organization may have a case management component for their frail elderly clients, while also making this program available to the community at large. This framework continues with services coordinated defined in terms of those provided by the organization only and community-wide services. An example would be a Department of Social Service caseworker coordinating all DSS services for a client versus coordinating community-wide resources for their client in addition to

DSS programs. The duration of case management also depends on the degree to which a system is open. Case management in a health care organization can stop at discharge from the system, three months later, or be ongoing as needed. Issues of financing are affected by the characteristics of the target population, the extent to which services are coordinated, and the duration of case management.

Many communities now have case management programs contracted or coordinated by the Area Agency on Aging. These programs have eligibility requirements that often exclude the less socially isolated, middle-income person. A sliding fee scale is usually used. Private case management programs are increasing, providing this service to the frail elderly ineligible for public programs. Private case managers provide the same benefits to clients and families as public programs; however, private case managers are free of restrictions in the scope of their practice. They may be limited, however, by the client's and family's ability to pay for extended services.

Finally, health care providers can assist their frail elderly patients and families by attending to good communication skills.

Toward this end, the American Association of Retired Persons (1987) has provided the following guidelines:

(1) Ask the patient and family to list symptoms and questions before a visit.
(2) Use open-ended questions.
(3) Avoid a formal, businesslike approach.
(4) Ask patients what name they prefer to use.
(5) Avoid medical jargon while giving clear explanations.
(6) State expectations of outcome.
(7) Summarize information.
(8) Provide positive feedback.
(9) Speak to the patient's and caregiver's level of vocabulary and understanding.
(10) Provide written information and direction.

SUMMARY

Multiple dependencies in activities of daily living and home management, cognitive impairment, social isolation, and low income are characteristics frequently found in the frail elderly. Family caregivers are mainly female, often middle-aged or older adults themselves, who express confusion and frustration in negotiating the aging services delivery network. They report a decrease in their sense of well-being and an awareness that their plans for the future have been changed. Many report a decline in physical health and stamina. Caregivers have had little education regarding their relatives' condition and probably no training as caregivers. Many do not freely choose this responsibility but rather are identified by family members or come forward themselves because there is no other alternative. Caregivers have difficulty meeting the needs of the present while trying to anticipate the future of an unpredictable progression of functional impairment.

A variety of community resources exist to assist family caregivers in meeting the needs of the frail elderly. Services vary with geographic location. It is important for health care providers to be knowledgeable about their service delivery system. Area Agencies on Aging, Departments of Social Services, and Community Mental Health Boards may be the appropriate places to start in exploring the extent of resources in addition to in-home nursing agencies and Public Health Departments. Support to caregivers through support groups and respite and day programs may be a significant factor in delaying institutionalization. Housing options exist to provide patients and families with optimum living environments or a continuum of care. Socioeconomic factors play an important role in the availability and procurement of services.

Health care providers need to collaborate fully with each other and human service providers to effectively assess and intervene with the frail elderly and their caregivers. Interdisciplinary geriatric teams provide the structure for comprehensive assessment, and case management continues this process with coordinated monitoring of services. There is a need for information, support, and recommendations for options in care; therefore clear communication is required when working with the functionally limited elderly and their caregivers.

REFERENCES

American Association of Retired Persons. (1987). *Older patients and you: Communicating with America's fastest growing patient group.* Washington, DC: Author.

Baldwin, D. C., & Tsukuda, R. A. W. (1981). Interdisciplinary teams. In C. Cassel & J. Walsh (Eds.), *Geriatric medicine: Vol 2. Fundamentals of geriatric care* (pp. 421-435). New York: Springer Verlag.

Given, B., & Simmons, S. (1977). The interdisciplinary health-care team, fact or fiction. *Nursing Forum, 16*(2), 165-184.

Horowitz, A. (1982, March). *The impact of caregiving on children of the frail elderly.* Paper presented at the meeting of the American Orthopsychiatric Association, San Francisco, CA.

Kane, R. (Ed.). (1988). Introduction (Case management issue). *Generations, Journal of the American Society on Aging, 12,*(5), 5-6.

Margolis, H., & Fiorell, J. S. (1984). An applied approach to facilitating interdisciplinary teamwork. *Journal of Rehabilitation, 50*(1), 13-17.

Michigan Department of Public Health. (1987). *Alzheimer's disease and related conditions.* Lansing, MI: Author.

Michigan Office of Services to the Aging. (1987). *Michigan needs assessment of 60 and over population.* Lansing, MI: Author.

National Center for Health Statistics (1987). D. Dawson, G. Hendershot, & J. Fulton (Eds.), Aging in the eighties, functional limitations of individuals age 65 years and over. *Advance data from vital and health statistics* (No. 133, DHHS Publication No. PHS 87-1250). Hyattsville, MD: Author.

Takamura, J. C. (1983). Health teams. In L. J. Campbell & S. Vivell (Eds.), *Interdisciplinary team training for primary care in geriatrics: An educational model for program development and evaluation* (pp. II-64-II-67). Los Angeles: University of California, Multi-campus Division of Geriatric Medicine.

White, M., & Simmons, W. J. (1988). Case management in hospitals. *Generations, Journal of the American Society on Aging, 12*(5), 34-38.

Part IV

THE MULTIDISCIPLINARY
ASPECTS OF HEALTH, ILLNESS,
AND DISABILITY IN LATER LIFE

Chapter 12

MULTIDISCIPLINARY PROFESSIONAL DEVELOPMENT IN GERIATRICS/ GERONTOLOGICAL HEALTH PRACTICAL SUGGESTIONS FOR PROGRAM PLANNING

ELIZABETH A. OLSON

The knowledge base in the field of aging and health is growing very rapidly. In order to provide the best services for older adults, geriatric and gerontological health care practitioners today must have ready access to information about advances in the field of health care and the implications of those advances for practice.

Most professionals endorse the concept of lifelong professional development or continuing education as one means to keep abreast of recent advances in the field. In the health field, continuing education is required to maintain licensure for nursing home administrators, nurses, social workers, and others. The purpose of professional development is to help health care practitioners acquire the knowledge, skills, attitudes, and behaviors needed to achieve the purposes of their professions and to improve their performance. Professional development continues throughout their careers and is a critical component of successful professional practice.

MULTIDISCIPLINARY ASPECTS OF PROFESSIONAL DEVELOPMENT

In the field of geriatric and gerontological health care, development of continuing education programs is of relatively recent origin. As more people live longer, interest in and new information about aging is appearing everywhere. New ideas, strategies, and research results are being published in hundreds of professional journals, popular magazines, and daily newspapers.

Information on aging emerges from such a great variety of sources because gerontology, or the study of the processes of aging, includes the multiple and interrelated changes that affect the biological, behavioral, and social aspects of later life. As such, it is considered to be multidisciplinary, drawing on the best science from a number of fields, each with its own body of knowledge, research methods, and professional organizations (Peterson, 1987, p. 1).

For those who provide professional health services to older clients, the multidisciplinary aspects of the field of aging--with its practical information from so many sources—can make it difficult to keep up with what is new or to decide which technique or strategy is best.

In this chapter, the focus is on the practitioner as learner in this multidisciplinary field. The purpose is to offer some guidelines and practical suggestions for those who plan and conduct short-term professional development programs on health and aging topics to help practitioners continue to develop and to improve their practices.

GUIDELINES AND PRACTICAL SUGGESTIONS

Health care professionals in the field of aging now have available to them a number of opportunities for increasing their knowledge, such as workshops, conferences, in-service programs, continuing education programs, health and aging journals, longer term educational programs, discussions with colleagues, and reflection on daily practice. The number of these options has grown rapidly as many colleges, universities, hospitals, and other organizations have recognized a need, expanded their offerings, and focused their content on specific areas in the field of aging.

One of the most popular formats for professional development programs is the short-term continuing education program. The need to maintain licensure has created many 1- or 2-day workshops that meet the licensing requirements and update people on new developments in the field. These programs usually are designed for mid-career individuals interested in improving or modifying their knowledge or skills.

Sork (1984) identified several advantages and limitations of this format. Its advantages include opportunities to learn a great deal in a concentrated program, to facilitate networking, to apply content immediately, and to refine problem-solving skills and get questions answered. Its major limitation is the time constraint, which may lead to information overload for the participant, to difficulty assisting a learner who has problems keeping up with other participants, to instructor fatigue, to difficulty correcting problems that arise during the session, and to difficulty providing individual feedback to learners.

By capitalizing on the advantages and taking into account the limitations, program planners can increase the likelihood that the program will be successful and produce positive outcomes. To begin planning a professional development program, the planner needs to do the following: explore trends in the field; determine needs; set goals and objectives; and plan, implement, and evaluate the program. Each of these areas is discussed below and practical suggestions are offered to facilitate program development.

Exploring Trends

The first step in planning a professional development program is to explore trends in the field and to identify a timely topic. In the field of aging and health services, trends may be observed in many areas, such as changing needs of clients, new legislation, professional journals, newsletters, conferences, and discussion with colleagues.

Once trends have been identified, the next step is to determine the educational needs of those for whom the program is being developed and to select a specific topic.

Determining Needs and Selecting a Topic

The primary consideration and the major planning challenge for professional development program planners is to respond to the goals, economic constraints, and training resources of the agency. In the field of aging, many agencies have limited resources designated for professional development; limited resources demand careful choices. Based on these constraints, the planner assesses professional development needs and identifies a specific program topic.

The identified needs will determine how the chosen topic is to be presented as a professional development program. The topic may be presented as one that provides basic knowledge about a particular need or it may meet practice-based needs, or both. Programs may focus on ideas that may be implemented immediately, or they may provide background knowledge about a new area. And, finally, programs may focus on basic information or may provide advanced or updated knowledge about a particular topic.

In terms of program focus or content, the two most common problems planners encounter are (1) the content is not relevant to the participants, or (2) the content is either too basic or too advanced. To avoid these problems, the planner needs to know the audience and, in particular, such factors as the background, learning abilities, interests, and attitudes of participants. The educational attainment of participants bears a significant relationship to the focus and instructional level of the program content. Those with more education and experience may benefit more from issue-oriented and advanced topic areas; those less experienced may benefit more from skills-enhancement programs.

The planner also needs to consider the multidisciplinary nature of topics in the field of aging. While the health care professional may be highly knowledgeable in a particular discipline, he or she may not necessarily also be knowledgeable in gerontology or geriatrics. It is more challenging to design a program that is multidisciplinary in focus than to concentrate on the needs of a particular discipline or profession. The planner may find it helpful to consult with professionals from the other disciplines involved when planning a program on a topic in aging that has multidisciplinary components.

It is the author's observation that, in general, today the most popular programs are those dealing with practice-related topics and special skills such as the assessment, diagnosis, counseling, or treatment of the frail elderly. Knowledge-based programs may be better attended when the programs are issue-oriented, presenting factual information within the context of major topic areas in which social problems appear, such as family caregiving, legal issues pertaining to the elderly, or long-term care issues.

Once the topic has been chosen, the planner will need to select a title for the program. The title should clearly describe the topic to be covered, be fairly short, target the audience (identify who should participate), and be appropriately worded for the designated audience (i.e., contain a minimum amount of jargon).

The next steps in program development are to set goals and objectives; plan the program; determine the budget; and promote, implement, and evaluate the program. These components may be discussed individually, but in actuality they overlap.

Setting Goals and Objectives

The overall goal of the program states its purpose, and the objectives describe the expected outcomes of the program. For example, if the overall purpose of the program is to introduce a new assessment tool to use with older clients, the objectives describe specifically how the participants will be trained to use the tool and what skills they will have learned by the end of the program. It is best to state goals and objectives in behavioral terms that can be measured so the planner can determine whether or not the program successfully achieved its goals and objectives.

Planning, Implementing and Evaluating the Program

Planning is the key to a successful program. The program plan describes the strategies, methods, and techniques the planner will use to impart information. Harris (1984) described four kinds of information the planner needs: (1) a list of the tasks that must be accomplished before, during, and after the program; (2) the amount of time needed to accomplish each task; (3) the resources and support staff needed to accomplish each task; and (4) the appropriate sequence for these tasks. There are many ways to gather and prepare this kind of information; for example, planning calendars are commercially available from office supply stores as well as other formats for timing and sequencing tasks.

A critical planning decision concerns the total amount of time that must be allowed for planning the program. The amount of time depends on a variety of factors, such as how long it takes to obtain the resources needed to implement the program, or when the instructor or speaker is available to present the program. The most common problem planners have is underestimating the length of time needed to plan and manage all the program tasks. The planner should expect delays and build in time for them. They are inevitable.

Determining the budget is an important part of the plan. Unless the planner has been given a blank check to cover program expenses, the costs of such items as presenter fees, supplies, refreshments, audiovisual rental, space/site rental, and promotion must be considered carefully. Two common problems encountered in establishing a budget are underestimation of costs and failure to anticipate all the costs involved. For example, the costs of items that seem small, such as those for refreshments or supplies, can add up quickly.

Program implementation begins with obtaining the presenter, selecting the supplies, and reserving the site. Identifying and selecting the best person to present the program is critical to its success. The planner should assess a potential presenter on the basis of recommendations by others in the field, and on the presenter's mastery of the content, sensitivity to participants' needs, and ability to cover the topic area in the allotted time. If the presenter will receive payment for the presentation, the planner should be certain to clarify what the fee will be and what it includes, such as preparation time, travel expenses, and meals and/or lodging.

Supplies, equipment, and handouts are aids that support the learning design. Selection of these items should be based on how much each will contribute to the objectives of the program. A film, for example, should only be used if it will directly help to accomplish one of the objectives. Other selection criteria include cost, availability, the presenter's skill in using the equipment, reliability, and readability.

The cost of supplies can add up quickly. The planner needs to determine whether or not such items as name tags, folders, duplication services, or special equipment will need to be purchased and to estimate the amount and cost. If audiovisual equipment (such as films, videos, screens, monitors, overhead projectors, or microphones) is needed, the planner needs to know where it can be obtained and at what cost.

The selection of the site usually is determined by the size of the group, the amount of rental fees, and any other needs the group may have. Two key dimensions of selecting the site are the tangible costs and benefits associated with it and its symbolic value. The tangible costs and benefits include rental fees and parking fees, as well as the comfort and convenience of the location. The symbolic value of a location may be as important as the tangible costs. Strong attitudes or beliefs, either positive or negative, may be associated with a particular site. Although conducting professional development programs at the place of work has many advantages, such as convenience, if the work setting has any adverse symbolic value it is better to select another place. Whatever site is selected, the planner should obtain space reservation and cost agreements in writing and confirm therm shortly before the scheduled program.

Promoting the program is an additional task that can have measurable impact on the program's success. The way in which a program is promoted may be as simple as announcing it at a staff meeting or as complex as marketing it to a broad range of professionals in the community. The function of promotion is to prompt participants to enroll in the planned program. In order to do so the planner will need to identify the target audience and determine how best to reach them.

When developing the overall plan and budget, the planner should determine what and how much promotion is needed, who will prepare it, and what the cost will be—including such costs as typesetting, duplication, postage, mailing labels, and direct mail costs.

Evaluating the program is the final step. Evaluation is critical to the long-term success of any professional development effort. Only through effective evaluation will the planner be able to improve and refine future programs.

There are many different evaluation models for professional development programs. The planner will need to decide what information is needed to satisfy evaluation requirements and how the results will be used. Categories of items to be evaluated most often include the design and implementation; participant participation; participant satisfaction; and participant knowledge, skills, and attitudes.

To evaluate program design and implementation, the planner may ask questions regarding the quality of the program such as the following: Was all the material covered? How much time was spent on each topic? Did the presenter follow the planned format? Did the sessions begin and end on time? Participants may be asked to judge the program based on such areas as the program content, the presenter's style, the physical facilities, and the cost. And presenters may be asked to contribute suggestions for changes to make before the next program. To formalize the answers, a questionnaire could be constructed to provide the kind of information needed to make the evaluation. This questionnaire should be completed by the planner, the participants, and the presenter.

CONCLUSION

This chapter highlights the basic components of planning professional development programs. Attention to each component should increase the success of the programs, while taking into account the planners' resources and skills and the needs of the practitioners for whom the programs are planned. The effort will be worthwhile if the knowledge and skills gained are translated into improved services for a growing older population.

REFERENCES

Harris, E. M. (1984). Planning and managing workshops for results. In T. J. Sork (Ed.), *Designing and implementing effective workshops*. San Francisco, CA: Jossey-Bass.

Peterson, D. A. (1987). *Careers in the field of aging*. Lexington, MA: D.C. Heath.

Sork, T. J. (Ed.). (1984). *Planning and managing workshops for results*. San Francisco, CA: Jossey-Bass.

AFTERWORD
Concerns and Their Resolutions
for Practitioners

ELIZABETH A. OLSON
ROSALIE F. YOUNG

The authors whose work is presented in this volume all have addressed critical issues for assuring the health and well-being of our elderly population. Recognizing that older persons will comprise an increasingly large proportion of our total population in years ahead, they have proposed interventions for practitioners in the health and human service fields. The suggested interventions acknowledge that these issues are serious at the present time, assume that they will become more pressing in the future and, most importantly, are addressed within the knowledge base that we presently have. Each author has detailed an action program salient to his or her field of practice that can be used by persons who serve geriatric clients or patients. Examining the concerns expressed by the practitioners and the interventions proposed, there are several commonalities. These are expressed in three themes, which are presented below.

INTERVENTION THEMES

Three overarching themes dominated the preceding chapters. One concerned the need for accurately defining the problem area or at-risk population needful of intervention. The second emphasized the importance of a partnership between the aged patient or client and the practitioner responsible for suggesting and/or implementing the intervention. The third and final theme focused on the need for individualization and flexibility of proposed interventions. Accurate definition of the problem to be addressed or the at-risk older person is critical. Without employing precise means of identifying the target population or correctly determining whether the individual is a candidate for the intervention, little will be accomplished. Clearly, some types of problems are difficult to diagnose and define. A notable example is the Alzheimer's disease patient. Guidelines do exist, however, and practitioners can avail themselves of materials that will make their diagnosis, definition, or identification of the jobs easier.

Establishing partnerships between aged persons and the professionals who treat or help them is essential. The gerontological and medical literature is filled with reports of asymmetrical patient-physician relationships that feature a set of physician-generated instructions offered to a passive patient; with practitioners who establish case management plans without determining client wishes and self-report of needs. Clearly, the older person in need of preventive or treatment services must be aware that professionals have noted that need, but the individual must be made a party to the plan for intervention. A symmetrical model must be established for intervention efforts to be successful, whether in dietary change, medication monitoring, or caregiver respite services.

Individualization and flexibility are additional concerns, if the proposed intervention is to be successful. The heterogeneity of the aged is now an established fact that only the most unaware persons do not acknowledge. Recognizing that there are major health and demographic differences in the older population, however, is not enough. Clearly, it is essential to plan different services for an 83-year-old woman living alone in an urban poverty area who can barely dress herself due to cardiac insufficiency, than for a 68-year-old man with a healthy spouse caregiver and a substantial income-investment portfolio who is severely arthritic but has no other health needs. It also is imperative to tailor the plan to psychosocial characteristics of the person. To illustrate, persons who have engaged in more active coping and

life-control behaviors may require different interventions that their counterparts. The practitioner planning interventions that can serve their older clients
and patients in an effective way must carefully consider these three areas of
concern.

SPECIFIC INTERVENTIONS PROPOSED
AND THEIR IMPLICATIONS

The authors of the preceding chapters addressed the needs of their geriatric
clients. Each proposed interventions that could alleviate the specific
problems they presented. Readers may note that there are implications for
most of the proposed interventions.

Robert Arking dealt with the basic question of longevity as it is linked to
modification of the aging process. He posed two types of interventions that
are potentially helpful in this regard: genetic manipulation and nutritional
intervention. Neither of these interventions, however, is presently available
as a technology practitioners can adopt.

Genetic manipulation is not feasible because our knowledge base does not
include the critical facts. Even if it did, the issue of medical ethics would
emerge as a major consideration. Advocating this type of genetic engineering
might represent eugenics for many people. Nutritional intervention to ensure
longer life for humans is untested. Scientific developments in biological
research show that severe caloric restriction appears to lengthen the life of
rats. Of course, whether human populations who cut their caloric intake to
approximately half the amount typical of adult diets can live longer has not
been shown. Indeed, since this particular intervention has not been tested
among humans, we, as practitioners, need to be cautious in proposing it. We
must be aware that food habits may have deleterious, as well as beneficial,
effects. Just as has been shown for many medications, sustained use can have
many unfavorable health consequences. It will take many years of testing for
us to determine what positive and negative results may unfold from severe
caloric restriction. Hence, practitioners need to carefully consider any scientific evidence that such practices can potentially lengthen human life.

Joseph Hess presents a series of health promotion and risk-reduction
practices that can benefit the aging person—as well as his or her younger
counterpart. All have been well documented as to their value in either the
prevention of serious chronic disease or slowing the progress of such conditions. While the literature has not conclusively shown that some health
behaviors, such as exercise or smoking cessation, are equally beneficial to

older and younger heart patients, it is clear that these practices are quite helpful to those with existing and emergent heart conditions.

An essential consideration is that there are two players in health promotion interventions—the patient and the medical practitioners. Neither can be assigned sole, or even primary, responsibility for achieving this goal. The life-style changes and the behavioral interventions that are detailed in this chapter all depend on patient and physician communication and on the cooperative efforts of both parties. Indeed, to decrease one's chances of succumbing to fatal disease or disabling conditions, the at-risk individual must be given medically relevant information on the appropriate intervention (for example, setting up appointments with cardiac rehabilitation facilities); then it is necessary to monitor the patient's progress with regard to health promotion and risk-reduction practices.

Martha Miller's chapter focuses on interventions that pharmacists, physicians, and nurses can fruitfully advocate that lessen the problem of medication misuse among the elderly. Among the most potentially deadly situations for the aged are those that involve the use of several prescription drugs to control multiple chronic conditions. The elderly not only are the major users of prescription medication, but they often take several medications and, in addition, are less able than younger persons to tolerate high dosages of these drugs. A most hazardous situation is set up and these polypharmaceutical aspects of health care for the elderly need the prompt attention of health providers.

The chapter presents several age-related changes in bodily functioning and how these allow medication buildup and facilitate medication misuse. Several specific strategies are proposed that involve education of health professionals and thorough knowledge of each patient's health and medication regime. Such strategies can be extremely beneficial in reducing the risk of medication misuse among the aged.

Rosamond Robbert presents an overview of the history of Alzheimer's disease and describes how Alzheimer's has become a household word. It is essential that professionals working with older persons and their families be familiar with the multiple issues associated with Alzheimer's disease and how they affect the patients, their families, and social institutions—especially the service delivery system. First, and foremost, is the need for an accurate diagnosis. Proper diagnosis is critical to management: many reversible conditions mimic a true dementia. Those conditions that can be treated may be overlooked if, as often seems to happen, a hasty diagnosis of Alzheimer's disease is made. A complete diagnostic workup is needed to accurately assess whether or not the older person actually has the disease.

In Chapter 5, Green and Bridgham discuss the issues and concerns involved in treating older alcoholic clients, including the prevalence of alcoholism; the criteria used to define alcoholism in the elderly; and its causes, diagnosis, and intervention strategies. One of the difficulties encountered by those treating older alcoholics is that of the compounding effects of alcoholism, normal aging changes, multiple chronic illnesses, and other problems. Our social values may deter our efforts to help someone who is both old and an alcoholic. Practitioners need to know what is fact and what is fiction regarding alcoholism in later life.

Cynthia Shelby-Lane's work addresses the serious problem of elderly abuse. Not only is this an area that often is overlooked, but health and human service providers who are aware of the magnitude of the problem may not know how to determine whether their older patients and clients are at risk for violent episodes. This chapter provides awareness of the prevalence of elder abuse, description of the at-risk individual, theories of abuse, and strategies for dealing with this in the practice environment. It can serve as a valuable guide to practitioners who encounter geriatric populations and want to know how to recognize and treat the problem.

The interventions proposed in the chapter on elder abuse increase the health provider's responsibilities in caring for the aged. It is no longer sufficient to just treat older patients. The practitioner must be prepared to ask questions about broken bones, burns, and injuries. He or she must not assume they are the result of sensory impairment, cognitive functioning declines, or old-fashioned carelessness. Injuries of the older adult must be approached in a similar manner to those the physician or nurse uses in assessing a child.

John Waller, using his extensive experience with health policy at the national, state, and local levels, has identified several critical areas of need. His focus on minority elderly is within the rubric of the general inadequacy of health policy efforts for older persons. This work links the economic aspects of health care for the aged through the Medicare and Medicaid systems with political efforts to regulate and restrict such care. His analysis of health policy includes implications for minority aged, as well as their nonminority counterparts.

Barbara Hirshorn contributes to the conceptualization of caregiving by introducing readers to the context of family care provision. Exchanges of assistance between generations—especially those between the frail elderly and their families—are presented using a holistic approach, that is, by looking at the many factors (such as demands on time and financial resources, as well as physical and psychological stress) that can influence family caregiving. Practitioners need to be aware of these factors as they assess the needs of the frail elderly and design ways to assist families. Who will provide the care and at what cost are issues that may need to be reexamined, with more innovative resolutions attempted.

Rosalie Young discusses the immense family implications of heart disease. A model of caregiving is presented that indicates the family context of health problems and the factors that influence recovery, caregiver strain, and adjustment to late-life health problems. Because heart disease is a major source of caregiving and can influence the speed of recovery of the heart disease patient, practitioners need to be concerned about how to predict which families will be able to provide appropriate care, or whether a family is of a personality type to provide the support needed. There is no simple or easy way to make such predictions. If such predictions are made at the time the patient is discharged from the hospital, it may be too late. There may not be time to conduct such an assessment while the patient is hospitalized. Becoming aware of the important role families can play in the recovery process can help practitioners to identify those supports most needed, and to move the family as rapidly as possible toward recovery.

In Chapter 10, Eva Kahana and Jennifer Kinney emphasize the need to bridge the research-intervention gap. The focus of their work is upon implementation of research findings for service providers concerned with caregivers. The past decade has seen an explosion of caregiving studies but few efforts to aid caregivers that are derived from sound models of caregiving strain. Without proposing interventions that are grounded in results of well-designed empirical studies, little may be gained. This chapter gives service providers a valuable set of guidelines for dealing with problems associated with adverse caregiving sequelae among care providers and patients alike.

Leon Schrauben describes the kinds of community resources and services that may be available to family caregivers to help their frail elderly family members maintain independence as long as possible. He stresses the need for coordination of information and referral activities. Because many frail older adults suffer from multiple chronic diseases and functional disabilities, it is difficult, if not impossible, for one practitioner to coordinate all the services that may assist the patient and the caregiver to keep the older person at home as long as possible. These services may make the difference between keeping the patient at home and institutionalization. Coordination and collaboration among practitioners seem to provide the best intervention supports. A concern, however, is that particular services may not always be available or convenient for all older adults. For example, those living in rural areas or in small towns may have access to a very limited number of support services. There is a need to devise ways to assist the geographically isolated.

Elizabeth Olson identifies the need for continuing education in the field of health and human services to the aging. The knowledge base in the field of aging is growing rapidly. The practitioner must have access to information about advances in the field of health care and the implications of those advances for practice in order to provide the best services for older adults. There are many opportunities available for professional development, such as health care and aging journals, continuing education or short-term training programs, and more lengthy educational programs.

CONCLUSION

In conclusion, there are serious issues that concern the health and human service needs of our growing aging population. The practitioners working with older people, the communities in which they live, and the politicians who control their health and functioning destinies need to recognize these problems and address them in a meaningful way. It is essential that they be constantly alert to new ways of more accurately assessing and meeting the needs of older citizens.

These chapters have, we believe, served a dual purpose. They have identified problems facing a society that has a significant number of older people, and they have proposed interventions that are timely, relatively simple, and may be quite cost-effective.

Some interventions will result in financial savings (for example, by focusing on preventive health to reduce the likelihood of the development of heart and other chronic diseases). Others can lengthen the life of many aged (for example, by alerting practitioners to drug toxicities and to persons at risk for violence). Still others can improve the quality of life of our aging population (for example, by facilitating interventions that enhance emotional well-being for both patient and caregiver).

We hope that practitioners will agree that their older patients and clients are worth the investment of time and effort these interventions require. We believe that implementation of such interventions will reduce the burden of illness and disability in later life and help refocus our society's attention on valuing the health and life quality of older adults.

INDEX

ABOUT THE CONTRIBUTORS

ELIZABETH A. OLSON is Education Director and an Assistant Professor at the Institute of Gerontology, Wayne State University, and an Adjunct Assistant Professor in the Departments of Sociology and Community Medicine. Since receiving her Ph.D. from Michigan State University, she has developed and implemented more than 250 short-term professional development programs for practitioners, covering many of the major topics in aging. Each year she directs a Summer Professional Development Program on Issues on Aging for health and human service providers. She conducted a Faculty Development in Gerontology Program, funded by the Administration on Aging, designed to train multidisciplinary faculty to teach gerontology to students in the health and human services disciplines, and administers a Graduate Certificate in Gerontology program for students enrolled in 20 different colleges and departments. She serves on 12 local, state, regional, and national boards and committees.

ROSALIE F. YOUNG, Ph.D., is a Medical Sociologist and Gerontologist. She is Director of the Health and Aging Program and Graduate Director of the Department of Community Medicine, Wayne State University School of Medicine. Dr. Young conducts research on aging and teaches medical and graduate students. For over 10 years, her research has focused on chronic diseases in later life, especially its personal and familial impact. Numerous publications and presentations have resulted from this work. Included are intensive studies of chronic disease prevention and medical management, caregiving to ailing aged, health problems of minorities, and the role of family support in mortality, morbidity, and psychosocial functioning. She currently is designing a community health promotion project for vulnerable populations, included the aged. This multidisciplinary effort involves the work of physicians, nurses, allied health professionals, social workers, sociobehavioral scientists, and community organizations.

ROBERT ARKING is an Associate Professor in the Department of Biological Sciences and a Faculty Associate of the Institute of Gerontology at Wayne State University in Detroit, Michigan. He received his undergraduate education at Dickenson College and earned his doctoral degree in biology from Temple University, where he was a NSA Predoctoral Cooperative Fellow. His thesis work involved the investigation of the mechanisms of gene action in the development of the geneticist's favorite animal, the fruitfly *Drosophila Melanogaster*. He continued his research in developmental genetics as a NIH Postdoctoral Fellow at the University of Virginia and as a Research Associate/Research Assistant Professor at the University of California, Irvine. Before coming to Wayne State, he also served on the faculty at the University of Kentucky.

JANET D. BRIDGHAM received her bachelor of arts degree from Radcliffe College and her M.S.W. from the School of Social Work at Michigan State University. She was employed as a therapist by the National Council on Alcoholism, Lansing Regional Area, before joining Nova Muir Green as a mental health therapist with the Ingham Eaton Clinton Community Mental Health Board. With Green, she implemented an Older Adult Substance Abuse Treatment Program and provided information, consultation, and education on older adult substance abuse treatment and issues.

NOVA MUIR GREEN received a bachelor of philosophy degree from Robert Maynard Hutchin's four-year college at the University of Chicago, a bachelor of arts degree from the University of Michigan, a master's degree from the Human Development Committee at the University of Chicago, and a M.S.W. from the School of Social Work at Michigan State University. She has experience as an instructor with the Office of Medical Education, Research, and Development at Michigan State University, and is currently a mental health therapist at the Clinton Eaton Ingham Community Mental Health Center in Lansing, Michigan. With Janet Bridgham, Green implemented a prevention, assessment, and treatment program designed to provide information and to assess substance abuse problems experienced by persons 55 years of age and older. She currently provides treatment to older adults with substance abuse problems and presents workshops, public presentations, and in-service education programs on older adult substance abuse problems and treatment.

JOSEPH W. HESS is a physician involved with teaching geriatric medicine for many years. The majority of his professional career was spent at Wayne State University School of Medicine. He was on the faculty of the Department of Internal Medicine from 1960 to 1974 and then was appointed Professor and Chairman of the Department of Family Medicine from 1974 to 1986. He organized and obtained funding for the first geriatric medicine fellowship at Wayne State University and was the principal investigator for a comprehensive health promotion/disease prevention research and demonstration project for healthy older adults in Detroit. Since joining the faculty at the University of Utah in 1988, he has been a faculty member in the Division of Geriatric Medicine with research interests in cancer screening, nutrition, and health care delivery. He also serves as faculty and research coordinator for the Geriatric Medicine and Dentistry Fellowship Program.

BARBARA HIRSHORN is an Assistant Research Professor at the Institute of Gerontology, Wayne State University. Cross-trained in policy analysis and planning, organizational sociology, and demography, she has focused much of her work on intergenerational (inter-cohort/inter-age group/inter-lineage generation) resource transfers. Specifically, she has examined private-sector behavior regarding the retention of older workers. She also has coauthored (with Eric Kingson and John Cornman) *Ties that Bind: The Interdependence of Generations,* a book that takes a life-course perspective on the intergenerational transfer of societal and familial resources as well as pointing out the pitfalls of using an "intergenerational inequity" approach to the distribution of resources in an aging society. Her current research concerns differences in labor force status and labor force behavior of middle-aged individuals who do/do not have concomitant parent care responsibilities and other ongoing family care needs. She is also collaborating on a series of analyses examining the intergenerational care receiving and sociodemographic structure of Americans 60 years of age and older, given a range of values regarding their health status and the availability of close kin for the provision of certain kinds of support.

EVA KAHANA is Professor and Chair of the Department of Sociology and Director of the Elderly Care Research Center at Case Western Reserve University. She currently serves as Director of Predoctoral and Postdoctoral Training Programs in Health Research and Aging. She has served as Chair of the Behavioral and Social Sciences section of the Gerontological Society of America (1984-1985) and is a member of the Council of Aging of the American Sociological Association (1986-1989). She is a recipient of a MERIT Award from the National Institute of Aging for the study of Adaptation to Frailty among Dispersed Elders (1989-1994). Her current research also includes a study of illness adaption of elderly heart attack victims and their caregivers, and a study of physician-patient communication in Alzheimer's disease. She has published extensively in the area of stress, coping, and health of the aged; late-life migration; and environmental influence on older persons.

JENNIFER KINNEY is an Assistant Professor at Bowling Green State University, where she coordinates the Graduate Certificate Program in Gerontology for the College of Health and Human Services. She earned her doctoral degree in psychology from Kent State University in 1987. Upon completion of her degree, she served as a Postdoctoral Research Fellow under Eva Kahana at Case Western Reserve University until she accepted her current position at Bowling Green University in 1988. Her interest in family caregiving began during her graduate work with Many Ann Parris Stephens. Her doctoral research involved the development of a scale to assess the daily hassles of caring for a family member with Alzheimer's disease. As a postdoctoral fellow she extended her interest in caregiving to include the formal network and other issues in caregiving. She currently is coinvestigator with John C. Cavanaugh on an National Institute on Aging grant investigating inter- and intraindividual differences in the stress-appraisal-coping process among caregivers to a family member with dementia.

MARTHA J. MILLER is a practicing pharmacist specializing in Geriatric Pharmacy Practice. Following completion of a Doctor of Pharmacy degree from the Philadelphia College of Pharmacy and Science, she completed a research fellowship in Geriatric Pharmacotherapy at the University of Georgia. She has been a member of the Wayne State University faculty and a consultant pharmacist for area long-term care facilities. She maintains an Adjunct Faculty position at Wayne State University and has published in the field of geriatric pharmacy practice.

ROSAMOND ROBBERT earned her PH.D. at Western Michigan University in sociology with a specialization in gerontology. She is currently Assistant Professor in the Gerontology Program at Sangamon State University, Springfield, Illinois, where she teaches a variety of courses in social gerontology. Her chapter in this book is in part based on a larger study titled, "The Medicalization of Senile Dementia: From 'Normality' to 'Pathology.'"

LEON SCHRAUBEN is supervisor of Medical Social Work and Home Care Planning at St. Lawrence Hospital, Lansing, Michigan, and instructor with the Center for Aging Education, Lansing Community College. He is a graduate of the School of Social Work, Michigan State University, and the Institute of Gerontology, University of Michigan. His interests include interdisciplinary geriatric practice and education, caregiving issues, and social work in health care. He has conducted workshops at state and national conferences and presented research on patient and caregiver expectations of health care at national meetings.

CYNTHIA SHELBY-LANE graduated from the University of Michigan Medical School in 1977 and completed a surgical residency at the University of Texas Medical School. She recently served as Chief of Emergency Medicine at Hutzel Hospital in Detroit, Michigan, where she was involved in the emergency treatment of older medical, surgical, and trauma patients. She serves on many boards and committees concerned with violence and its aftereffects. She has addressed many physician groups about professional responsibilities associated with treating violence victims. She also prepared the film, *Wasted Dreams,* about the consequences of violence for black youth.

JOHN B. WALLER, JR., is Chair of the Department of Community Medicine and Associate Professor of Epidemiology at Wayne State University. He is Codirector of the Maternal and Child Health Institute and Director of the Center for Prevention and Control of Interpersonal Violence at Wayne State University. He served as Director of Public Health for the City of Detroit from 1978 to 1987. During his years of public service he contributed to many health policy decisions that affected the lives of older citizens. He serves on local, state, and national boards, including the Executive Board of the American Public Health Association. He has been particularly interested in the health problems of minorities, and his work in this area has been acknowledged by Louis Sullivan, Secretary of Health and Human Services.